PHILOSOPHY AND ETHICS OF MEDICINE

SBN 443 00572 9

Printed in Great Britain

PHILOSOPHY AND ETHICS OF MEDICINE

MICHAEL GELFAND
C.B.E., M.D., F.R.C.P., D.P.H., D.M.R.

Professor of Medicine, University College of Rhodesia;
Honorary Physician, University of Birmingham

Foreword by

SIR ROBERT AITKEN
M.D., D.Phil., F.R.C.P.

Vice-Chancellor, University of Birmingham

E. & S. LIVINGSTONE LTD
EDINBURGH AND LONDON
1968

To

JAMES MONTGOMERY

O.B.E., M.D., F.R.C.S.(Edin.)

" . . . a very perfect practiser "

FOREWORD

THE scientific content of medicine grows and changes fast. This puts an increasing intellectual strain on medical students, on their clinical teachers, and on all other practitioners. The social function of medicine is possibly changing too, but much more slowly. As a topic of study it is apt to be crowded out of the busy minds of students and teachers. What purpose does medicine serve in society? How must doctors behave in their personal relations with patients and with other doctors, and what values must they adopt, in order best to fulfil that purpose? Those are questions much less discussed than problems of drugs, operations, or chromosomes. Yet they are equally important, and if they are not discussed the behaviour may change and the values slide, disadvantageously, before we are aware of it.

In the chapters of this book Professor Gelfand explores these matters of behaviour and values. He traces them historically and then describes them as he sees them today, mostly among practitioners in the British tradition but with a sideways glance now and then at the African witch-doctor. He does not preach and he does not lay down rules, though on controversial issues he is perfectly clear about what he himself does and why. He does not praise the good and blame the bad, but lets the ideas of good and bad emerge from the story of how doctors do in fact behave. With its personal flavour, and its almost conversational style, this presentation is better than a text-book, for it challenges the reader to exercise his own judgment in the situations it describes. There are behind it thirty years of unique practice in Central Africa.

With this book in their hands, the medical students of Salisbury, Rhodesia, will need no formal lectures on medical ethics; students elsewhere may find the same. For all of them, and for their seniors too, Professor Gelfand offers something which is far from dogmatic instruction, but close to the ideal mode of university teaching, whereby the pupil shares the experience and this discourse of a master.

ROBERT AITKEN

Birmingham, 1968

02975

PREFACE

ALMOST all doctors with whom I have discussed this point have admitted that they were given little instruction on the ethics of medicine. Indeed in many medical schools the student receives no formal course of lectures on it. Yet none of us can practice medicine without meeting an ethical or moral problem almost every day. Not infrequently we observe or hear of errors, some serious, committed in the course of practice, which could perhaps have been avoided had the doctor been warned of the risks he was likely to run before he engaged in medicine. It is not enough to leave such matters to his common sense.

Many of our medical schools provide no instruction in medical history. This I consider a sad lack, for an understanding of our past is one of the best means of instilling the medical recruit with respect for what we have achieved and a sense of pride in and regard for our aspirations. From this knowledge grows a truer desire for and insistence on correct medical behaviour.

Not only do we need to know the greatness or virtues of any sphere of activity in life but also its drawbacks and the weaknesses that may appear. Although, on the whole, the contributions of medicine are emphasised, we have to take a realistic view, remembering that the profession is handled by human beings and therefore weaknesses are liable to arise, which, in turn, develop into difficulties and disappointments. This applies not only to medicine but to every field of human endeavour. And so my object is to try to give a true picture taking into account both the good and the bad.

With a deep regard for medical history I next found my mind turning to its philosophy and I began talking to my house officers about medical logic and ethics. One in particular, Dr. Alan Cohen assisted me greatly in argument and gave up many nights to discuss the questions that were occupying my thoughts. When the Medical School in Rhodesia began, the Birmingham Medical Faculty sponsoring it agreed that I should deliver a course of formal lectures in medical history.

Side by side with these developments was the close contact I had had for many years with the witchdoctor and his medical approach. Through him I was able to study at first hand his pseudo-scientific practices with his largely spiritual concept of disease. The contrast in the two methods of practising medicine caused me to think deeply about the philosophy of medical practice. All this presented a challenge that I felt must not be left unanswered. This book is an attempt at an answer.

I earnestly hope that this book will meet the needs of the medical student and practitioner and provide a basis for further argument and debate.

I have already thanked Dr. Alan Cohen for his valuable aid. I am also deeply grateful to my friends Dr. V. N. Barlow and Dr. Brendan Berney, who spent so much of their time in discussions which helped to make this book possible, and to Professor Bernard Blackstone who helped me both in discussion and correction of the manuscript. It was always a pleasant experience to discuss the philosophy of medical practice with him. Dr. R. S. Roberts, a medical historian, took a personal interest in my work and I would like to record his assistance. I also owe a special word of thanks to the Hon. Mr. Justice B. Goldin for his helpful suggestions and understanding.

Mr. A. Harrison, the medical librarian of the University College of Rhodesia, kindly helped me to find many of the articles on the philosophy of medicine. Mrs. H. P. Payne, my secretary, made my task all the more pleasurable by her enthusiasm and careful assistance.

MICHAEL GELFAND

University College of Rhodesia,
Salisbury, 1968

CONTENTS

1

INTRODUCTION

I CAN claim that I have been immersed in the active conduct
of medical practice for over 30 years. I can claim, too, to
understand the members of my profession, and equally that
I have treated man in the many afflictions to which human
flesh is heir. I have seen him make a complete recovery. I
have been present when he has been taken away suddenly
and I have experienced the feelings of those around him, sad
at the thought of his passing. I have often been thanked for
my part in helping a patient to good health, and at times I have
suffered the cold looks of the family when it was thought that
I had not done all I could for his recovery. I have known
success and also disappointment. I have seen patients of all
social grades from the highest to the lowest in the land. I have
witnessed man in his success and in happiness and equally in
his sorrows. I have served him and watched all his vicissitudes,
his inconstancies, his loves, his hates, his addictions, his prejudices—all have been my lot to share.

In all the triumphs and failures I have shared my experiences
with my colleagues. I have worked with physician, surgeon
and family doctor. In this association our relations were
mostly smooth, but I can recall times when a colleague chose
to be difficult or when perhaps he felt that I had done something that displeased him. There were also occasions when I
was annoyed at the attitude of others towards me ; at times I
was disappointed with their outlook towards the public or
reaction to certain social or educational matters. But through
all my service in medicine I have adhered to the tenets of my
calling and followed closely its teachings.

It is understandable, therefore, that there were times when
I was inwardly troubled by ethical problems that arose and

1

by my own attitude both to the public and my colleagues. Often my conscience was torn by what I had done or refused to do. I felt keenly the anguish on the faces of those I could not help. At other times there were particular issues in which I personally was not concerned, but I was aware of them and perplexed by the problems they involved. I well recall the occasion when the unmarried daughter of a leading citizen fell pregnant and how a doctor—a very staunch Roman Catholic—took part in arranging for the termination of her pregnancy. I could not understand how such a religious man could forgo his principles. Yet there was a young girl with her life before her placed in this predicament. For long my mind was worried by the rights and wrongs of this case. On one side was the suffering of the father and his daughter and on the other the foetus—a living thing. Few would deny that there was great sympathy on either side. And then as my practice grew, I found myself facing the same requests from married and unmarried women. Each time there was a plea for help I had to summon up all my courage not to let down the principles of my profession. It was a hard battle. Repeatedly the thought would come, " there are so many people in the world, does it matter if there is one less?" And so our minds are plagued. Who can forget the eyes of the girl sitting opposite pleading for help, unaware of how one's soul was tortured. And yet I could not see my way clear to assist unless there was a strong medical indication that the life of the mother would be threatened.

I have often met patients, frequently amongst the highest in the land, who resorted to unorthodox medical procedures when one of their family was afflicted with a serious disease. Time after time I was asked to agree to the trial of some ' quack ' remedy. Frequently I was amazed at the existence of yet another spiritual healer of whom I had never heard. Many of them seemed to be carrying on a lucrative type of practice treating incurable growths and other fatal complaints. When death threatened a family its members were quick to learn where to contact these practitioners. What was I to do? What was may attitude to be? My profession forbade me to work with them. Under such circumstances when I knew there was nothing more my profession could do for the patient I turned a blind eye to what was happening. I have even consented to the employment of such a practitioner at the request of the family when I could offer no more help to those for whom I was so distressed. Would I have been justified in refusing to extend a friendly hand to the ' quack ' who was being asked to try to help the patient?

These are some of the problems that have perplexed me. I have frequently wondered whether the cures claimed at Lourdes were all falsely based. I personally cannot claim that I have seen a miracle. When one of my patients has contracted an incurable disease and there has been irrefutable proof of its existence I have never seen the affliction leave the person. Yet we read of wonderful cures brought about not only by religious bodies, but also by witchdoctors, spiritualists and others. I have given much thought to the medical methods employed but have satisfied myself by clinging to the scientific approach. Even amongst my own profession I am told of amazing treatments given in Europe to make the old young again. I recall seeing a very able and successful business man who was greatly troubled by headaches. In desperation he flew to Switzerland where he saw a doctor (the fee ran into three figures) and all he was advised was to drink three glassfuls of hot water every night. And what is more the headaches completely left the patient. I say to myself, ' This is surely psychological '. But for all that, deep in my consciousness the thought persists, 'Am I absolutely sure?'

It is not strange working as I do largely among Africans that I come into close contact with the witchdoctor, who practises so extensively amongst the Africans throughout this continent. He still wields enormous influence and the African masses still cling to his methods of practice. Instead of finding him greatly feared by his public, I discovered that he is revered. On the whole his people preferred his opinion and treatment to mine. I was regularly asked to allow my patients to leave hospital so that their relations could take them to consult a witchdoctor. Whenever I thought the patient would be definitely harmed by leaving hospital I did all I could to dissuade the family, but very often I was unable to change their minds and the patients were discharged. I could not know their ultimate destiny or how many recovered. At times I felt so strongly about the threat to their lives by leaving hospital that I insisted on their remaining, but at the same time I could not be really sure that I was right in this. I was invariably worried about the ethics of what I was doing. Although I was confident I was right and had the scientific method of approach to back my opinion, I often wondered whether by chance I was wrong for I could not be absolutely certain that the desperately sick man would not benefit more from his own sort of 'quack practitioners'. I suppose many doctors have had these qualms. I often think of an African maid who worked in my house for a number of years. She always seemed to enjoy good health until about two years ago when, at the age of 45, she became very ill. Her body was swollen. She was desperately sick with a nephritic disorder and her blood pressure was high. I looked after her in hospital and despite a stormy passage she made a good recovery under my treatment. And then, after a few days, she seemed to have a setback. She became rapidly worse and vomited repeatedly. I was worried, but felt that as she had improved before she would respond again. However, she made little progress and then to my consternation her husband asked if he could take her to a witchdoctor. I pointed out that this was the wrong thing to do and although I admitted how ill she was, I informed him that I was confident that she would recover under my care. However, he insisted and took away the sick woman. I was certain her condition would deteriorate. To my amazement she returned to my home three weeks later apparently fully recovered, wanting to start work again. I was so impressed that I asked to see the witchdoctor to find out what medicines or herbs he had employed. He came to my house, a fine-looking African from Mozambique. He explained what he had done. He attributed her illness to someone who had bewitched her, but would not say who this person was. At the same time he had given her certain roots to take by mouth to counteract the evil. She has been very well ever since then. It may well have been that she was about to recover when she left hospital. It may have been that my drugs had upset her and that when they were discontinued she could be expected to recover. This is one of the very few cases in my experience in which recovery could perhaps be attributed to the witchdoctor's efforts.

Throughout my years of active practice I have always had an unhappy conscience on the charging of patients. To charge or not to charge? Was it right to send a bill to a man whom I knew could not afford this amount? If I did not charge him would I embarrass the practitioner who referred him to me? Would the patient be ill-disposed to him because he had sent an account and the specialist had not submitted one? I recall a doctor once explaining that he could not send me work if I did not charge the patient. The more I thought of his point of view the more I realised that he had a case. Again there was embarrassment to the doctor if my account was very small or moderate and his large because of his more frequent visits. The patient might think he was overcharging. As the years went by I came to see the points of view of both sides. Just like any other citizen the doctor needs to earn a comfortable living and at the same time the patient should not be financially embarrassed over his illness.

In all these years I have had much to do with my colleagues. I am fond of the medical world which seems to lead its own sort of life closely bound up with its daily problems, and although I did little service on any committee I was always in close touch with the matters that concerned us all—our rights of practice, arguments between doctors or bitter feelings to one another for various reasons. I tasted the acute rivalry that exists between medical men and was often puzzled as to why it was there. But it existed. There were differences between general practitioners and specialists and between salaried and non-salaried doctors. I saw how medical cliques could arise and how jealousy became rife between individual doctors. These feelings were strong, even in academic circles and among the full-time staff of the hospitals it was very real and few doctors escaped its bite. Although I have always tried to avoid friction and I am sure my medical colleagues did too, difficulties arose and seemed unavoidable. They were sometimes followed by bad relations and a bitterness that was never forgotten. Entry to hospitals, appointments and vested interests are all real and part of the human make-up wherever we are. Whether the doctors are practising in a small town or village or in a large city community, the same occurs. At times the problems seem mostly of an economic nature—a threat to the doctor's income or a struggle to maintain his appointments. Sometimes the profession, or rather the majority of the practitioners in a place, appear to close their ranks to prevent newcomers gaining entrance to the hospital, or even from settling there. I remember when I first arrived in Rhodesia after my postgraduate training in England hoping to start a practice, I was staying in Bulawayo at the time. The advice I received was that I should go to Salisbury, where there was a shortage of doctors. And when I went to Salisbury to decide whether to settle there, various medical men informed me that there was far more scope in Bulawayo.

A doctor's life is a hard one and yet there seems to be a feeling amongst all of us that we are as one: we belong to a sort of guild although we have no real trade union and many doctors do not belong to a medical association. But we have much in common: we are exposed to the same dangers and seem to be of one company. I have learnt to admire the hardworking qualities of most doctors who labour long hours and are available at any time. They do not care how many hours a day they work when running busy practices. I cannot understand the fuss made about short hours by people in industry. Yet the non-medical world seems not to consider this aspect as it affects the medical practitioner.

I think the examples mentioned above show good reason why a study of the philosophy of medicine is necessary. Many members of my profession are interested in the philosophy of medicine, many write on the subject; indeed they have been writing on it for centuries. Certainly all doctors think about this matter even if they do not define it precisely in their own minds. No one can practise medicine without talking about it. It is true that most thoughts and discussions revolve around what might be regarded as the ethics of medicine, which is an important aspect of its philosophy but there are other aspects to be remembered.

The philosophy of medicine must embrace all questions relating to the life of man in the universe and to all matters that threaten or upset him. I would regard it as including all that appertains to the purpose or aim of medicine or what it stands for, not only in the eyes of the medically trained person but in those of all people, for the doctor is only one figure, albeit an important one, in the conduct of medical practice. Therefore the issue which arises at once is the epistemology of medicine or, in other words, a consideration of the basic principles or theories of medical knowledge and the validity of these principles. For example what are the basic principles of the various types of medical knowledge? Which type is valid? Are there any with no validity?

It is presumed that from the very beginning of his existence man has tried to help the sick. Some have prayed to a deity for this help. Others have studied the movement of stars, others again have prescribed herbs. Each method embraces a theory of knowledge. Epistemology also includes the reason advanced for the success of a particular theory of knowledge. Experiment in the scientific world, for instance, is an important item of this approach.

In any concept of the philosophy of medicine it is essential to debate the ethics of medicine, that is what might be regarded as right or wrong in accordance with our standards. Clearly this is an important aspect of such a study, but not the only one. It concerns the correct, or what is believed to be the correct attitude of mind of the patient to the doctor, as well as that of the doctor to the patient and, last but not least, the conduct or behaviour of medical men among themselves. A third component of the philosophy of medicine concerns the effect or impact that the practice of medicine has on the community or the public as a whole. We have to judge where medicine has been of service to mankind and where it has rendered a disservice. This we must regard as the social aspect of the philosophy of medicine.

In this study an attempt is made to give a picture of medicine, as I see it, although, being a doctor myself, I may be accused of bias. In the expression of these views my purpose has been to put forward the ideas of people as a whole, explaining the attitude of man to medicine and how the knowledge of medicine can best be brought to the sick, ailing or those in need of help.

2

MEDICAL EPISTEMOLOGY

THE MEDICINE OF HIPPOCRATES, GALEN AND HARVEY

THE NEED for medical care must be as old as man. He enjoys feeling well and when confronted with pain or some other disorder of function—whether indigestion, pain in his chest or headache—he tries to find out what is disturbing him. He may fear too that his life is threatened and that unless his symptoms are relieved he will die. Therefore the possibility of death turns him to seek medical aid and it is this very realisation that one day he must die that distinguishes him from the animals. He knows that there may be help at hand which can remove the threat and so he must find it. A young child or infant in pain is much like an animal in that he tends to resist the attentions of those who try to assist him.

The appearance on the scene of a medical person who could devote himself to the relief of the sick began probably in Ancient Egypt and China somewhere about 2500 B.C. At the time of the Old Testament, however, nearly 6000 years ago, there is no description of such a person and the healing of the sick was apparently entrusted largely to priests. Thus in the days of the Old Testament, disease was probably regarded as being of religious origin, that is, the cause of an illness was linked with sin. Through prayers and supplication God's forgiveness could be obtained and the sick one allowed to recover. In God lay the power to cure, or even to raise the dead. Yet we know that the ancient Hebrews stressed the value of cleanliness and the frequent use of washing. Perhaps these instructions were given with good reason. Water tended to cleanse and could perhaps remove the taint of evil from a person's body. Certainly in African society today it is believed that an individual should avoid touching or coming into physical contact with a stranger in case he is endowed with evil. In Biblical times too a large number of dietary laws were introduced, many of which are still adhered to by Jews today. But in the original writings there seems to be no direct implication that the underlying motive for their introduction was the preservation of health. There is a temptation to argue that these dietetic restrictions have this aim. Thus a pig infected with *Taenia Solium* would be a danger to health if consumed as food. Why, then, was beef allowed when this might be similarly affected? While it is possible that these rules were designed to provide a basis for good living, it should be stressed that there may have been other reasons for them. We know that in Africa today every clan has its own totem and this animal may not be eaten under any circumstances by that particular clan.

Even long before the Hebrews a predominantly spiritual cause for disease was probably the universally accepted concept. Paleolithic and neolithic man very likely attributed disease to deities. When the famous Abbe Breuil studied the Bushmen rock paintings in Rhodesia depicting the animals upon which man then depended entirely for his existence, he postulated the theory that the person who led the services at these shrines was indeed the first " doctor " although his main duties were sacerdotal. Standing before the rock with the hunters who were shortly to go out in search of the much coveted game, and pointing to the pictures, this leader invoked the spiritual powers to bless their hunters and give them success in their chase. This man, endowed with the ability to contact these powers, presumably could be consulted also when any one of the clan was afflicted with an illness. At the same time Man looked around in nature for measures which he thought would keep him in good health. He tried cleansing his body with water as well as practising certain dietetic avoidances, selected entirely on an empirical basis.

Two or three thousand years or even longer before Hippocrates, men with a medical interest were attempting to treat disease and pondering on whether it could be attributed to the outside world. It seemed to them that something came from outside, possibly from afar, and entered the body. And so once this influence was known, illness could perhaps be avoided or an attempt made at cure, provided these cosmic forces could be tapped. We are told that Hermes Trismegistus, a figure of great wisdom and philosophy, was the first to give the world a new medical outlook. Some say he was a person in Egypt, whereas others have chosen to link him with the deity Thoth. Others again hold that the teachings of others were incorporated in the Corpus Hermeticum. We can regard Hermetic beliefs as mostly philosophical or metaphysical. Hermes looked to the firmament above—the *supra*—containing the heavens with the sun, moon and constellations, the light and influence of which gave rise to life below (*infra*). Therefore Hermes enunciated his great principle of " supra ut infra." What is above in the outer firmament of the macrocosm is the same on earth below with its products of this influence, plants, animals, and man the microcosm. " That which is inferior is as that which is superior, and that which is superior is as that which is inferior." Although the macrocosm was created out of nothingness, yet everything that was not perishable, such as the earth, was created by the influence of the macrocosm and was composed of three elements, the trinity of mercury, sulphur and salt. The perishable things in the microcosm (man with his soul) were made of four elements, earth, water, air and fire, each of which arose from the trinity of mercury, sulphur and salt. Thus long before Hippocrates we find the birth of the idea of chemistry or, more correctly, alchemy, and Hermes has been called the father of the chemical art (Blackstone, personal communication). He formulated the doctrine of correspondence according to which all the stars send out influences, reminiscent of our present day cosmic rays. Every child born comes under the influences of a particular formation of stars which happen to be present within the zodiacal house at that particular time. This formation is known as the conjunction of the planets.

In accordance with Hermetic belief every species of plant or animal in the macrocosm was nurtured through the influence of its own star in the Zodiac at its birth and so if this conjunction in the macrocosm could be discovered and also therefore the corresponding plant in it, treatment could be instituted to assist in the recovery of man (microcosm) who for some reason, had lost its beneficial influence. Therefore the patient's star had to be found and then its corresponding sub-lunar substance with which to treat that individual.

Probably about 2600 B.C. medically inclined persons first began to devote some of their energies to healing. It is not known for certain where they started but there seems to be some evidence that in the first stages they were diviners and exorcists who did not necessarily confine themselves to medical matters, but were consulted about other problems as well. This was perhaps the first breakaway from the priest or minister of religion. When man in the Neolithic period had exterminated the game and thus threatened his own existence he discovered in the Fertile Crescent, between the Euphrates and Tigris rivers, how to obtain food from the soil. He turned to farming and at the same time reared domestic animals which supplied his main source of protein. As he obtained his food from the soil he became aware of the seasons of the year, the sun, the heat, the rain, the wind and the water—all of which helped him to exist. Here in the Fertile Crescent, possibly for the first time, the turning of his thoughts to the different cosmic deities ultimately gave rise to some of the great religions of the world. He felt that there must exist in Nature powers which could be tapped or utilised and so there came into being men and women who claimed that they were specially endowed with the gift of knowledge as to how these powers could be contacted, or that they could interpret certain omens released by these powers or spiritual forces. Not all people had this gift of knowing what lay behind the movement of the stars, the changing shape of the moon or indeed the changes in the appearance of the liver of a sheep when its abdomen was opened. These knowledgeable people were the diviners who were consulted in any matter of concern to any person. Special medical cults sprang up, the best known perhaps being that of Hermes or Thoth in Egypt or that of Asclepius which had a large following in Ancient Greece and Rome. By going to one of his temples and contacting its priest, the sick person would be visited by the spirit of Asclepius (usually in the form of a serpent) whilst he slept and through this spirit he could be expected to recover. There was yet a third popular method of treatment closely linked with the belief in a spiritual cause of disease. Not only were there good forces in Nature upon which man could draw, but there existed evil or dangerous spirits of divers kinds, demons and devils pervading the whole universe, including a person's own home. Terrible though it was to conceive, another individual could be the seat of such an evil source of power and its influence could be passed on to an unsuspecting person by the mere touch or glance of that individual and in this way he could be struck down with a painful death. Thus amongst these ancients arose people who were believed to be able to heal by removing or exorcising the evil from the sick person. This was often done by placing a goat in contact with the patient and causing the evil to pass into the animal (hence the term " scapegoat "). Not only was the exorcist able to purify the patient but through his divining powers he could point out the guilty individual or witch who could then be removed from society by force or death to cleanse it of evil. What was happening at this time differed little if at all from what we meet in Africa today. Once this concept of a mystical cause of death is accepted there is no need for the patient to be examined or his symptoms to be discussed. All that the witchdoctor has to do is to learn from the occult powers what spirit, good or evil, is responsible for the trouble and what is necessary to propitiate it or in the case of an evil spirit what procedure the exorcist has to adopt to cleanse the patient.

Then in about 2500 B.C. there was a significant advance when man in his search for cures detected hidden virtues in plants. Egypt seems to have been the centre of this activity. There herbalism was evolved and developed to a far greater extent than in any other country, as is revealed in the papyri. Side by side with the spiritual or magical procedures adopted by diviners and exorcists was established the use of special herbal cures. At first this latent power in plants was considered to depend on the principle of symbolism by which like produced like effects. If taken by a woman in need of milk the plant with a milky sap was believed to induce a good flow of milk in her. But the virtue of plants was not only seen in symbolism. *Similia similibus curantus,* as these plants were used by the physicians of Egypt and neighbouring lands men began to find by experience that certain good results followed. Through experience and careful observation arose the school of empiricists.

From a study of the papyri Sigerist (1951)[1] shows that Egyptian medicine had a common origin in magical, religious and empirical elements. At this early time, about 2500 B.C., Egypt could claim both physicians and magicians employing methods both religious and empirical in concept. We know the physician interrogated his patient and then examined him. We also know that he looked at the urine, stool and sputum. The Egyptians even conceived of a kind of circulatory system of vessels originating in the heart. Along this they believed air, blood and tears were carried. Although, just as the witch-doctors in Africa today, the physician of Egypt may have appreciated that a number of symptoms collectively constitute a particular pattern, yet, for practical purposes, a disease meant a symptom. Thus cough, pain etc. were treated as diseases. But for all this, from their incantations and placa-

---

[1] Sigerist, H. E. (1951). *A History of Medicine,* Vol. I. London, Oxford University Press.

tions of the healing god, it is clear that the magico-religious element constituted an important aspect of the practice of the doctor of this period. It is probable that in any severe and threatening illness an appeal was made to the gods, and sacrifices were offered as well to propitiate an offended spirit. At the same time careful consideration was given to the possibility of an evil spirit having taken hold of the sick one in which case some form of exorcism was attempted.

Thus by about 2000 B.C. there existed in the Middle East and lands nearby physicians who spent their time with the sick and thought in terms of curing them. Even though the real understanding of disease was a long way off at least during this period of divination men believed there must be a specific cause for disease and if this were removed the patient would recover.

With the practice of many forms of divination and exorcism, as well as herbal therapeutics, medical theory must have been in a confused state. It is generally believed that the next advance in the concept of disease took place in Greece, but this is probably not so, as similar ideas were evolved in India and China much earlier. In these lands men were thinking already of disease as starting within the body itself, due to some incompatibility or alteration in its constitution. This concept can best be described as metaphysical. Instead of spirits or demons destroying the person from without it was believed that the normal health of the individual was being disturbed by a new agent developing within the body itself. Who exactly started this train of thought is a question irrelevant to this chapter. Even in Greece it was probably Aristotle (384 B.C.) and not Hippocrates (460 B.C.) who spoke of the body humours. Aristotle claimed that all things in Nature came from one of four elements—air, water, fire and earth— and that when any pair were united one of four qualities resulted. As a corollary to this metaphysical argument it was propounded that the humours or liquids formed in the body by the union of these elements gave rise to blood, phlegm, yellow and black bile. Any malmixture or excess of one over the rest caused a person to become melancholic, sanguine, phlegmatic or choleric.

We have already seen that the early Chinese and Indian civilisations had a similar " chemical " concept of disease. The early Chinese also spoke of the five elements—wood, fire, earth, metal and water which encompass all the phenomena of nature. Everything on earth belongs to one or several of these five categories. From at least 2800 B.C. we learn of another example of metaphysical theory for disease. It postu-lated a metaphysical union of two great principles—the male and positive Yang and the female and negative Yin. The human body was composed of Yang and Yin organs. The Yang one was characterised by heat or warmth and the Yin one was cold and dark like the female. The heart and liver were Yang organs whereas the kidneys and spleen belonged to the Yin variety. Good health followed a proper balance between the two principles and sickness resulted from an imbalance of them. Moreover, the Yang-Yin hypothesis depended on a combination of the five elements in the body —earth, fire, water, minerals and wood. As the heart was Yang any disorder of this organ was associated with a red forehead, whereas a red nose indicated that the spleen was at fault. We are also told that the ancient Chinese physicians paid special attention to the pulse, which was taken in eleven different places besides the wrists and was divided into three parts, the inch, bar and cubit pulse, each of which indicated a different internal organ. Prognosis was determined by the strength or irregularity of the pulse.

The Chinese also introduced in prehistoric times treatment by acupuncture, which consists of inserting fine needles into specific points in the skin. Whilst acupuncture might have been explained on the erroneous concept of a disharmony between the Yin and Yang forces of existence, the measure based on much experience may have been effective just as physiotherapy might be. Ancient Chinese physicians claimed to help to cure by acupuncture any disorder which resulted from a disturbed function of an organ. When diseased an organ would reveal itself by producing pain along a defined path, called a meridian, which was specific for that particular organ. For instance a disordered heart would be recognised by pain referred typically down the left arm. According to this hypothesis the energy of life flows through these meridians and the continued health of an organ (of which there are twelve all-important organs and therefore twelve meridians) depends on the unimpeded flow of Yang and Yin influences. When a needle is inserted into a particular point the balance of energy is re-established in the disordered organ.[1]

Evidence is now available that the Hindu held not altogether dissimilar views. Keele tells us that 500 years before Hippocrates physicians practising in India spoke of three main forces —sensibility, anger and stupidity—which were the basis of physiology, and of three " humours "—wind, bile and phlegm. They believed sickness followed disproportion of these humours. For instance, if wind rushed round the body it shook and developed spasms similar to those we associate with epilepsy.[2]

However, it is true to say that although physicians in Egypt, China and India had evolved some of the Hippocratic procedures, they were largely adopted by the Western world mainly through the influence of the Greeks. During the long Byzantine period Arabian physicians studied the Greek texts and established their medical schools in the countries under their dominance. They kept alive the flame and prevented medical knowledge from degenerating into the magico-spiritual beliefs which predominated in the earlier period.

Hippocratic teaching moved away from the attribution of illness to spiritual causes and instead concentrated on the body itself, the symptoms and signs of disease and how best to

[1] Mann, F. (1962). *Acupuncture, The Ancient Chinese Art of Healing.* London, Heinemann.
[2] Keele, K. D. (1963). *The Evolution of Clinical Methods in Medicine.* London, Pitman.

handle these with a predominantly empirical or rational treatment.[1] Alcmaeon of Athens, more than anyone else, influenced the Hippocratic school towards empiricism. He stressed that good or normal health depended on a proper balance between certain opposites and therefore disease followed when these were improperly proportioned. The new Grecian outlook regarded with disfavour the earlier schools in which the metaphysical approach predominated. It tried to be more practical, discouraging religious dogma. The men of Cos experimented on what we might call the natural history or course of a disease so that the doctor armed with this knowledge could predict its outcome. Nevertheless the metaphysical element remained strong for many centuries, especially with regard to diseases in which experiments failed to find a treatment based on accurate observations and long experience.

Hippocratic writings reveal a clear appreciation that diseases follow a constant pattern with distinctive clinical features and a special prognosis for each. This was a great advance over the spiritual school which paid little or no attention to the existence of a special syndrome for each disease, as it believed that the particular spirit affecting a body could produce any symptom in any part of it.

We owe much to Claudius Galen, about 100 A.D., who advanced the concept of a disorder in the body leading to disease and stressed that it was essential to examine the body in order to find out what might be the matter with it. He accepted the metaphysical theory of the four basic humours which he believed passed through the body by a sort of circulation. Man inhaled the vital spirit into the lungs from where it reached the heart. It now mixed with another spirit, the natural spirit, which came from the liver. The newly-formed product was sent up by the ebb and flow in the blood to the brain where this newly-formed spirit, called the animal spirit, was distributed along the arteries and nerves to cause motion

---

[1] Jones, W. H. S. (1948). *Hippocrates with an English Translation*. Heinemann, Harvard University Press.

and initiate sensation. Galen's hypothesis was accepted not only by the profession but also by the Roman Catholic Church, which saw in it a true explanation of the inhalation of the vital spirit or animus from God. Galen's concept of the transmission of the vital spirit through the body remained the accepted dogma until the first proof of the blood circulation in 1628. Until Harvey's momentous discovery, medical practice still followed a mixed or confused procedure with the Hippocratic or Galenic approach on one hand and the spiritual or magico-spiritual concept on the other. Men often practised both. Treatment had little which could be described as rational. Asclepiades (c. 110 B.C.) seems to have started the hypothesis of methodism in treatment. He taught that there were only three characteristics of all diseases which influenced treatment. One set of diseases resulted from constriction or relaxation of the pores, whilst the others were due to a mixture of these two. Thus the methodists treated with relaxing or constrictive drugs, depending on whether the body needed constriction or relaxation.[1]

It is not surprising that in all this uncertainty there was yet another group of physicians who treated disease simply by trial and error based largely on experience. These were the empiricists. With this approach and imbued with the Hippocratic method they tried to further knowledge and practice. Many of their advances were small, yet they reveal how the physician of those days tried to look at the body for an explanation of the disorder. In the opening centuries of the first millenium, for instance, doctors used the matula in which the different levels of the sediment of the urine were noted. The level of the sediment was thought to correspond to the part of the body affected. We now know that this hypothesis was incorrect, but it is of interest to observe that the physician of this period was looking to the urine for evidence of what might have gone wrong within the body. This search for a

[1] Poynter, F. N. L. & Keele, K. D. (1961). *A Short History of Medicine.* London, Mills & Boon.

clue to the disease certainly became more realistic when Paracelsus in the sixteenth century suggested that by adding chemicals to the urine special changes would occur in it, so giving rise to clues as to what disorder of function had occurred in the body. Paracelsus was ahead of his time for scientific chemistry had not come into being; it was still largely a practice of alchemy, a pseudo-science. But clearly men were beginning to think hard and were knocking at the door of truth.

The Hippocratics looked for clues, indeed for any clue that might be revealed by the body. They began to think that disease would be recognised by a study of the mouth or of the excreta from the bowel and bladder. The urine varied in colour and in amount in disease. After Galen there followed the Byzantine period when the Arabs concentrated on these forms of physical examination. By the fourteenth century the practice of urinary examination reached its height. The matula was used by the best physicians and one large Italian type was divided into three parts, depicting the head, viscera and genitalia and the sediment of colour appearing in one of these zones indicating the part of the body affected.

The Hermetic influence continued to exert itself and could claim many adherents in the medical profession right up to and even after the time of Harvey in the seventeenth century. The doctrine of the great Paracelsus himself was a mixture of both Hermes and Hippocrates. In essence this school embraced both the metaphysical and empirical approaches to medicine. The sixteenth century Paracelsus wrote widely that the sun, moon and all the stars and planets were in man because the human body attracted heaven. He accepted the hypothesis that man was composed of the four elements. He wanted the doctor to learn every aspect of knowledge in case each branch might contribute to an understanding of human disease. Therefore he believed that a good doctor should understand philosophy, astronomy, alchemy and ethics. Paracelsus taught that the light in man came from the firmament with all its constellations and from the heavens he acquired wisdom, art and reason, thus setting up an invisible ethereal body. On the other hand, he postulated that the second influence emanated from matter itself—the visible material body—and this was responsible for eating, drinking and all things connected with flesh and blood. Thus he maintained there were two opposite bodily wants depending on the influence from the heavens and from the material body itself, and in this way conflict or excess could develop.

Well into the seventeenth century leading physicians of the time still accepted astrology as a method of diagnosis of disease ; they believed that movements of the celestial bodies influenced the human body. Universities taught astrology in the fifteenth and sixteenth centuries. Anaemia, we are told, could be explained by this " science " or metaphysics. A person lacking in the influence of the planet Mars showed a deficiency in the Martian element, i.e. iron, and so iron was prescribed.

When man was well these influences and the parts of the body were considered to act in unison. The sun exerted vitality, Mercury the power of communication, and Venus harmony. An imbalance of these influences was followed by disease. Thus in the metaphysics of astrology the cause of an illness and its probable outcome were determined by the doctor without any physical examination of the body.

The Hippocratic method replaced the spiritual conception of disease largely because of the influence of chemistry and more precise knowledge of disease. The discovery of the circulation of the blood followed, then the evolution of physiology and later the appreciation of pathology. As Hippocratic medicine gained strength the spiritual and metaphysical schools played a secondary although still influential role.

First the Renaissance era came with Galileo's more precise measurements of time through his clock with a pendulum. This principle was accepted early in the sixteenth century by the celebrated Italian physician Sanctorius who introduced his simple pulsilogium to measure the pulse rate. Another simple yet significant advance was Galileo's thermoscope, modified by Sanctorius to reveal a rough estimate of the body temperature. This was the forerunner of the clinical thermometer of the eighteenth century.

Most important of all, perhaps, was Leonardo da Vinci's influence on medicine through anatomy due to his insistence on accuracy of description of every anatomical structure. He was followed by the great Andreas Vesalius, who demonstrated in his *Fabrica* that Galen's anatomical descriptions mostly applied to animals and not to man. Other Italian anatomists such as Realdus Columbus, and Michael Servetus, a Spanish theologian and doctor, postulated the existence of the pulmonary circulation. All these discoveries occurred at a time when the influence of the Church reigned supreme and with it the theories of Galen. The final proof of the circulation of the blood was made in 1628 by William Harvey.

What did Harvey's discovery mean at first? It made very little difference for about 150 years. He knew that the heart pumped blood through the body and that it must carry some vital elements to the different tissues. Treatment was not further advanced by the discovery as the theory of the vital spirits of Galen and the humours of Hippocrates was still generally accepted. There was still much to learn before the significance of Harvey's discovery could be appreciated.

Nevertheless, there was an ever increasing number of independent discoveries which helped to unravel some of the basic mysteries and produced a deeper realisation that disease originated within the body and that each illness had its own characteristic features. This concept was first put forward by Thomas Sydenham (1624-89), often referred to as the English Hippocrates, who claimed that disease could be compared to flowers, each with its own distinctive features. Then Robert Boyle (1658) showed that an animal and a burning candle both died when placed in a confined space. Both used some of the air. What was this vital substance they utilised? About 125 years later Joseph Priestley prepared a gas from mercurius calcinatus, in which candles burnt more brightly. He thus revealed the vital part of the atmosphere which Boyle had found essential for life and in 1774 Antoine Lavoisier, appreciating the full significance of Priestley's discovery, called it oxygen. Men now began to demonstrate other substances like amino acids in the circulation. Lavoisier's contribution on oxygen was taken up in other fields by Justus von Liebig (1803-1873) who showed that the protein, fats and carbohydrates were broken down inside the body into amino acids, glycerol and glucose respectively. Claude Bernard (1813-1878) demonstrated how the blood was concerned with the transport of glucose and other substances absorbed from the gastrointestinal tract into the portal veins, whence they reached the liver where the glucose was converted into glycogen. Chemistry had come into its own and assumed a new significance in the nineteenth century.

What caused special symptoms of disease to appear? Whence did they originate? Man had performed autopsies before, but no-one linked symptoms with the morbid changes seen in the organs after death until the appearance of Giovanni Morgagni's book, *On the Sites and Causes of Disease*. This contribution linked morbid anatomy with the patient's symptoms and stimulated the next remarkable objective approach to the understanding of disease. It will be remembered that Galileo introduced the telescope and compound microscope. Defective as it was then, this microscope was used both by Malpighi of Italy (1628-1694) and Leeuwenhoek of Holland (1632-1723) to observe the minute structure of organs and tissues. Robert Hooke (1635-1702) introduced the concept that all tissue was composed of layers of cells. The microscopic study of tissue cells had begun. It is not surprising therefore that the German pathologist, Rudolph Virchow (1821-1902), introduced cellular pathology in 1858 as the obvious sequel to Morgagni's changes seen with the naked eye. Morgagni's observations of damage to the internal viscera started with the revolution in clinical methods which aimed at linking the patient's symptoms and signs with the morbid lesions he and others had begun to describe. In 1761 Leopold Auenbrugger introduced percussion and not long after Rene Theophile Laennec (1781-1826) produced his elementary stethoscope with which he listened to heart sounds. By this time the emphasis and concentration of medical thought were directed almost entirely on the body itself. Nature was generous in the release of her secrets and man was now able to benefit from her revelations.

When Leeuwenhoek demonstrated the existence of bacteria and animalcula with his microscope no one associated them with disease. They were just another phenomenon of nature. But in 1836 Schwann showed that putrefaction was caused by these organisms. Until then it was thought that life was created by dissolution of tissue. It was thought that maggots that gathered on dead flesh developed spontaneously—the hypothesis of spontaneous generation. Schwann suggested that they did not arise *de novo*, but from eggs deposited there by flies. Louis Pasteur followed up these observations and convinced the doubting world that these organisms could produce disease and that there was a microscopic cause for many illnesses. Robert Koch enunciated the criteria upon which an organism could be accepted as a cause of disease and ushered in the era of bacteriology. Disease had a cause which could be handled and controlled. And from Pasteur's experiments there followed Joseph Lister's antiseptic methods of treating wounds in 1865 when a new era in surgery was born. All advances in medicine have confirmed the scientific approach and with its acceptance medicine has progressed further and further from its early concept of a spiritual reason for the cause of disease.[1] Today there is virtually no support for the metaphysics that held sway before the days of Harvey.

Modern physiology may be said to have had its beginnings with Albrecht von Haller (1708-1777) who was interested

[1] Poynter, F. N. L. & Keele, K. D. (1961). *A Short History of Medicine.* London, Mills & Boon.

mostly in the functions of the central nervous system. He held that nerves are mixed, partly motor and partly sensory. Other workers were stimulated to follow this train of thought. Charles Bell (1774-1842) of Britain observed that when the anterior roots emerging from the spinal cord were touched the muscles of the back of the animal concerned " convulsed ", whereas this did not occur with the posterior roots. Next Francois Magendie (1783-1855) of France cut the posterior nerve roots of a limb and noticed that all sensation in it was lost. In 1830 with the demonstration of the reflex arc, by which sensory nerves link with motor nerves in the spinal cord, modern neurology was born.

When Galvani (1737-1798) published his findings on his so-called animal electricity which flowed down the legs of his dissected frogs he did not realise that he was opening a new field in clinical medicine. From his observations arose our realisation of electrical activity in the brain and heart, thus enabling us to lead off these currents from the surface of the body and so detect abnormalities in them.

We see, therefore, how medicine has altered over the years with each new advance in science. At first Hippocrates looked critically at the patients and then turned to evaluate what he had perceived by his senses. Then interest turned to the organs, first the larger ones and thereafter to a minute study of the tissues and cellular structure of the viscera. We have now entered into the era of the cell with its nucleus and cytoplasm. Objectivity is the slogan of the followers of the Greek founder of our craft.

From the epistemological history, it might appear that there are numerous theories to explain medical knowledge, but three basic principles underlie all of them. They are the mystical, sensory and rational principles.

The *Mystical Principle* refers to knowledge obtained from the mind or as it can also be called the " pure reason " of the mind, the " intuition " or the imagination. No objective sensory evidence is necessary to confirm its validity. The origin of this knowledge comes only through the mind of the one who claims to know but he cannot prove his knowledge in a scientific manner. Examples of types of epistemologies containing this principle include the spiritual, magical, religous and metaphysical.

The *Sensory Principle* embraces the knowledge acquired through man's senses. Objective sensual evidence is used whereas mystical type data are excluded. Examples of types of epistemologies containing this principle are the scientific and empirical.

The *Rational Principle* includes the knowledge obtained through man's reasoning power. It is that knowledge which explains and connects together the basic elements in the theory. This principle is found to a greater and lesser extent in all types of theory for medical knowledge, i.e. spiritual, magical, metaphysical, scientific and empirical, mystical or sensory principles make up the main elements of the theory, and the rational principle ties up all and makes it into one rational whole.

In many cases the theory contains both mystical and sensory principles, and usually one dominates the other. But whatever the proportion of mystical to sensory principles, the rational principle is always present in varying degree.

The success of present day medicine is due to the scientific theory which consists purely of the sensory and rational principles. The mystical principle is disregarded. The sensory principle has been enhanced by the invention of instruments and machines (thermometer and stethoscope) which give most accurate objective sensory data. The rational principle has greatly benefited the theory by being responsible for the adoption of the experimental method and helping to evolve the numerous " brilliant inferences " that have led various men to discovery.

Briefly, the scientific theory can be said to consist of:—

(1) Observation of objective sensory evidence.

(2) Finding a relationship in the evidence.

(3) Making a rational hypothesis from this relationship.

(4) Conducting experiments to support the hypothesis.

(5) When the support is sufficient, a general law is proposed concerning the relationship. This law is subject to changes when further evidence makes this necessary.

(6) In practice, the law will or will not be confirmed by results from its application.

3

THE PURPOSE OF MEDICINE

THE aims of medicine are to help to restore the health of a person and to maintain it by preventing it from deteriorating or being attacked by disease. This leads us to consider medicine from two aspects, the curative and the preventive. Many people regard the function of the doctor as being merely that of cure or alleviation of pain and suffering, but that is not a true assessment of his duties as he is equally concerned with preventive measures. This is not a modern concept as, for centuries, the medical man, whether he pursued the Hippocratic form of practice or accepted other more spiritual cults, has always attempted by one means or another to prevent sickness, trouble, disappointment and tragedy. The witch-doctor of Africa, like the medical man of any other race, appreciates that it is better to avoid disease than to rely only on curing it. He is well versed in the innumerable charms and talismans intended to prevent disease and prescribes them daily. Many people, no matter in which of the various religions they believe, are convinced that prayer helps to keep men well in a world full of uncertainty. No one knows what the morrow will bring and this uncertainty creates fear.

Others have defined the aims of medicine in much the same way as I have. For instance, Reisler (1963)[1] sees them as an attempt to maintain health, prevent or cure an illness, alleviate pain and prolong life and productivity. Berman (1962)[2] says much the same, " Our members have never lost sight of their primary objective—the care of the patient; to cure if possible, if not to relieve discomfort (mental and physical) and to

[1] Reisler, S. (1963). *J. Int. Coll. Surg.*, **39,** 617.
[2] Berman, J. K. (1962). *Archs. Surg., Chicago,* **86,** 691.

prolong life." A French writer, M. S. Houdart,[1] said in 1836 that a physician's prime duty is to effect a cure.

It may be argued that the object of cure or prevention of disease is designed to bring about the ultimate happiness of the individual. In this objective there is perhaps a false claim since the doctor is not so much concerned with the state of happiness of the patient as he is with removing the cause of the ailment. If he sees a patient with typhoid fever his purpose is to find the cause and prescribe a treatment. Admittedly the patient will be happy when this is achieved, but only in the limited sense, pleased that he is well again. Happiness has a wider application. A person who is unhappy over his financial position may at the same time develop an acute illness. The doctor cures his illness with the specific remedy. He and the patient are pleased that he has recovered from the illness, but the patient's general feeling of unhappiness will persist as long as he is financially embarrassed. It is hardly the function of the doctor to balance the patient's finances and help him rid himself of debt so that he will be happy again.

The aim of a sick person is to rid himself of the morbid changes of which he is aware are in his body. For this he seeks aid but not necessarily from an orthodox medical man. He may prefer an unorthodox opinion such as that of a spiritualist or an osteopath. As is often the case, he may consult his doctor first, but if he finds that he is no better for his treatment he may turn to a faith healer. Thus the purpose of medicine is not the prerogative of the doctor or indeed of the medical profession. The medical profession cannot claim this but it believes that its method and approach are the correct and proper ones and that other methods are unreliable and may be dangerous. We have to remember that the object of the sick person is to be restored to health and that he is prepared to try any cult or group whose object it is to cure, provided of course, he has confidence in its claims. Every type of healer

[1] Houdart, M. S. *Hippocrates*. The Loeb Classical Library (1948), p. 17. Translated by W. H. S. Jones. Heinemann, Harvard University Press.

claims cures and all have the same object. The aim of the medical profession to cure or help is no different from that of those who present an unorthodox methodology.

In spite of overwhelming objective evidence that the doctor's approach to disease is correct and that he therefore fulfils the purpose of medicine by instituting a variety of remedial procedures, the unorthodox medical world makes the same claims without conforming to the criteria of scientific cure. The orthodox medical profession can prove how damage to a particular organ is followed by certain well-known effects. No other medical cult can do this. We know how an ulcer in the duodenum gives rise to a typical picture of pain before or after meals and that this discomfort is relieved by eating or taking an alkali. We know that such an ulcer may bleed when a blood vessel is eroded or perforates into the general abdominal cavity and we can demonstrate with great regularity the ulcer on X-ray and also at operation. We know that such an ulcer is accompanied by the secretion of an excess of free hydrochloric acid. There is hardly an organ in the body about which we cannot make similar statements. In other words, the approach of the medical man is based upon a knowledge of structure, function and symptoms and signs which follow when a lesion develops in the particular organ.

Once bacteria could be isolated and cultured and their properties and actions determined with repeated regularity, scientists were able to introduce vaccines containing the killed bacteria, which, when injected into the body, could afford protection against specific organisms. But this was not all. Men realised that there were organisms even smaller than bacteria which could not be recognised with an ordinary microscope and in 1923 it become possible to examine these bodies or viruses with the aid of the electron microscope which is fitted with special image intensifiers. Today at least 150 virus diseases have been recognised and again, using the same method of treatment as with bacterial disease, we have practically eliminated poliomyelitis. We realise that disease is not only caused by bacteria or viruses. There are many in which the cell of the tissue starts to proliferate to reproduce its own kind. This type of growth, of which there are various forms, may spread to other parts of the body as well as being invasive and destructive locally. We refer to such a tumour (the carcinomas and sarcomas) as being malignant. Thus we are aware of a large number of tumours which can be recognised by microscopic examination. They often produce well-known clinical features which help us to recognise them. Further, we know much about their sensitivity to radiation and, after confirming the diagnosis, can determine whether to use this form of treatment or whether in other instances excision offers the best chance of cure.

We have also learnt much about those diseases that are inherited and passed on through families. They generally follow a well-defined pattern and course. There is nothing magical about it. The study of genetics is coldly objective and adopts the true scientific method.

We can observe the features of a disease in a certain organ and note its constant repetition in other individuals. The same can be said about treatment. Many diseases respond in a particular way to a certain drug and this is generally repeated each time a patient is treated for this disease. We can quote the instance of myasthenia gravis which mostly responds to the drug prostigmine. The muscle weakness disappears almost dramatically when it is given, but once the effects of the drug begin to wear off the weakness or myasthenia returns.

The medical approach may be defined as conforming in essentials to the Newtonian principles followed by all scientists. It seeks the truth based on repetitive experience.

I prefer to regard the object of medicine as being to heal or help the sick and prevent an individual from becoming ill. To heal or help the sick is perhaps closer to the meaning of medicine than to preserve life. If the object of medicine were simply to heal the sick, could this always be achieved? We must admit that doctors often fail to cure a man suffering from congestive heart failure, for instance, although he can be kept relatively well on drugs for many years. In such cases we have not healed but helped to relieve the weakened heart. So we would be closer to the real meaning of medicine if we accept that its aim is to heal the sick by whatever means appear reasonable to the doctor, or, if full healing cannot be achieved, to lessen the severity of the illness so that the patient can continue to live. Thus the ultimate object of medicine is to cure or relieve the complaint of the patient by recognised procedures according to the code of Hippocrates.

It follows from this that medicine must be concerned with preserving life or avoiding any measure which attempts to end it before its time. At all costs the sick person should be kept alive and this raises the problem evident to everyone including perhaps the patient himself, of an inevitable end which may be very painful as well as protracted. It can be argued that by helping the sufferer to die, a merciful release is procured. Provided it can be established that there is no possible hope of recovery, whether the patient suffers pain or not, or even if there seems to be good reason for it would euthanasia be inconsistent with the principles of medicine. By taking this action the doctors are tampering with the principle of preserving life even if it is certain that the end is inevitable. Once it is accepted that euthanasia is inconsistent with the principles of medicine, the doctor is not entitled to hasten the painful and inevitable end that is approaching. He must continue the treatment that will give the patient most relief.

The medical profession aims at preserving life when the life of the individual is affected by disease. This is in keeping with the aims of medicine, but the medical profession is not more concerned than people in other walks of life with the loss of life which occurs through wars or even through everyday occurrences such as accidents. In fact medical men have taken their part in military campaigns for centuries. If they come into contact with anyone injured or sick, friend or foe, they can be relied upon to relieve the distress, but as a body they are not opposed to the principles of war, which they do not consider in conflict with the aims of medicine. The medical profession is not made up of conscientious objectors.

Recently the question has arisen whether a medical super-intendent can direct doctors on his staff on resuscitation. Members of the public protested against such a directive being given. The hospital superintendent's directive advised against resuscitation in old people or those with serious chronic disease, including malignancy. Personally I believe that this is a matter for the doctor treating the case who should make the decision, as each case would depend on its own circumstances such as the extent of damage to vital viscera and the likelihood of restoring the afflicted organs to a state of reasonable and useful normality.

We might go even further and observe that medicine only aims at the preservation of the life of man. Medical research may involve the sacrifice of animals through planned experiment. It takes the view that man is all important and therefore it is justifiable to perform experiments on living animals with the hope that man will benefit. The basic aim of medicine is to help man and not other forms of life. This does not mean that the medical profession does not appreciate the need of avoiding cruelty to animals. In this connection we are reminded how in the latter part of the nineteenth century, when there was rising opposition to animal experimentation in England, Queen Victoria sought the advice of Lister who insisted that it should not be stopped. In his reply to Her Majesty he explained that vivisection experiments were essential for the progress of medicine and he pointed out that the world at large, although so meticulous about preserving the lives of these animals, did not object to killing men and women at war.

What is understood by the health of the individual? This is difficult to explain but perhaps we may regard it as a sense of well-being in a sound body which is able to discharge its functions. A feeling of well-being is not enough. A cripple

3

lying in bed may have a sense of well-being but as he cannot walk his lower limbs cannot discharge their function.

It may be argued that a person may have valvular disease of the heart or even diabetes mellitus without being aware of any ill-health. I have not uncommonly seen patients who, on being examined for fitness for the civil service, were found to have damaged heart valves and yet they were totally unaware of this. It is true that later symptoms of heart failure would have ensued. There are many people walking about with a high blood pressure who seem to enjoy perfect health. Can we say that they are in good health? We might reply that any person with an abnormal blood pressure cannot be said to have good health yet we know that it is possible for any such person to live a long and useful life without any limitation to his activities. Nevertheless we cannot regard a person with an abnormality of heart, brain or lungs as being in good health even though he has no complaint. Therefore I prefer to regard health as that state of well-being or feeling of soundness by an individual provided no physical defect or abnormality is found in his constitution on examination. I must confess I am not certain what exactly we mean by *normal*. Normality defies exact definition for no two people are completely alike. There are so many variations in the body and yet individuals with them enjoy a sense of well-being. Normal means the usual state or condition of man. Medically speaking normal refers to that state of a body organ or tissue which maintains or ensures an individual's general feeling of well-being or does not threaten to disturb it.

I have purposely avoided specifically referring before to well-being. It is customary to mention both the physical and mental state, intimating that the two are distinct or apart, one dealing with the functions of the body (*soma*) and the other with those of the mind (*psyche*). I am not convinced that this distinction exists for the brain has a function like any other organ of the body, such as the liver, heart or kidney. And whilst I admit that the function of the mind is very important yet it is as necessary for the well-being of the individual for all his bodily functions not to affect it. Just as we cannot have a sense of well-being if the mind is affected, we cannot enjoy this feeling if the liver is out of order.

As already mentioned, in his desire to rid himself of this suffering the patient sees nothing wrong in going to a faith healer for aid. The medical profession claims that its approach is the right one and that other methods are unreliable and may even be harmful. Whether the profession believes that it and only it knows the true method of healing I cannot say. No doubt many doctors—perhaps the bulk of them—believe this in all honesty, but there are some who are more tolerant and admit that there may be some virtue in certain of the cults that have not received recognition by the profession. I personally believe in the Hippocratic approach but I cannot deny that there may be other methods. Many Christian doctors, when faced with illness themselves or in their wives or children, pray earnestly for a speedy restoration to health. The Christian believes that prayer can effect a remedy.

Despite overwhelming objective evidence that the doctor's approach to disease is correct and therefore he fulfils the purpose of medicine by instituting a variety of empirical and successful remedies, the unorthodox medical world remains unmoved and puts forward its claims even though they do not conform to the criteria of scientific cure.

Is the patient harming himself if he prefers to seek the aid of a spiritual healer? Is the Christian scientist committing an offence against his body by resorting to practices which may harm him when there is a scientific method of treatment available? I remember being asked to carry out an autopsy on a European man, sixty years of age. He was a Christian Scientist who became ill with what appeared to be malaria. But he refused all treatment and died. I have seen many Africans die because they did not receive early treatment. They died of diseases like pneumonia, malaria, typhoid fever, for all of which we have very high cure rates. Knowing this cure rate with specific remedies I believe that most of these people would have survived had they presented earlier for treatment. Many diseases which were often fatal in former days, such as diphtheria, leprosy, tuberculosis and syphilis, have all lost their sting through modern advances. We can say the same about the management of childbirth. Because of these advances the incidence of puerperal fever has become much less. So I can tell my patients with good reason that when they contract a disease it is in their interest to see their medical practitioner early so that a diagnosis can be made and the appropriate treatment instituted in good time. I stress the importance of consulting a medical practitioner first, because I doubt whether the non-medically trained person is in a position to reach a proper opinion as to what is wrong. Because of the many cures that can be effected today, there is good reason for the medical man to be consulted in the first instance.

Let us assume that a patient has first consulted his doctor for intractable headaches, migraine or a neuralgic complaint and the various remedies tried by him have failed to effect a cure. Is it wrong for the patient to seek help outside the profession? Provided a doctor has diagnosed an ailment for which the medical profession has no specific cure, in my opinion, the patient is justified in going elsewhere. If the profession cannot help him, can it demand that he should not seek aid from outside its ranks? The doctor is not obliged to suggest that the patient consult an unorthodox practitioner since he believes that his methods are based on false premises, but, if the patient makes this decision on his own, he should have no qualms about it. On the other hand, a Christian Scientist who believes only in prayer and not in orthodox methods of cure is harming himself when he is ill, since he may easily be suffering from a condition for which orthodox medicine can rightly claim a good remedy. It is most important for every person who feels ill to consult his doctor first to make certain that he is not suffering from a remedial disorder before he resorts to other measures. If the medical profession fails to restore him to his normal state of health he is then free to try unorthodox practitioners even though his doctor cannot aid him in seeking heterodox advice.

Even if a doctor holds strong views against unorthodox cults not accepted by the medical profession he should conduct himself in a dignified manner. He should avoid using terms like " quacks ", " impostors ", " charlatans ". Instead he should take a realistic view of the situation and whilst he does not accept the teachings of these unorthodox cults he should show tolerance towards them.

We can claim that medicine is responsible for the great increase in population in the world today, but can it be said that this is of benefit to man and has the profession done a disservice to the world? I do not believe that control of population is basically a concern of the doctor. He serves man by preserving his life in accordance with the aims of medicine. But at the same time he realises that in some countries, where economic factors are such that they may not be able to support the many people who have to be fed, the phenomenal increase in population may soon threaten healthy living. From this has arisen a desire in certain countries to advocate smaller families. Again I maintain this is not really a problem for the medical man. He is there to save life and fight disease. If a couple elect not to have children in their family it is not his concern. Even if more babies are born into the world than is good it is his duty to help all those born into it. It is true this might be easier and more effective if there were less overcrowding and less demand on food resources. If a husband and wife wish to use contraceptives, if the doctor so desires he can advise them. He is not destroying life in this way for conception has not yet occurred. His attitude towards contraception may be influenced by his religious principles, but this is a personal consideration rather than a medical one. But once conception has taken place it is wrong for the doctor to destroy its product, unless, of course, there is a real risk to the life of the mother. He would be contravening his ethical code if he destroyed the living foetus merely because the world would be better off for fewer people and thus fewer mouths to feed.

The purpose of medicine implies that a person is ill and therefore requires help either medical or surgical. Therefore if someone is not ill it would be wrong to operate and so Lord Brock in a letter to the London *Times* (3 Feb. 1967) warns against supporting legislation in favour of abortion for social and not medical reasons. As a doctor he is opposed to this and stresses that it is not acceptable to the medical code to perform an operation on non-medical grounds. At present it is not legal and a surgeon " who does an operation for other than medical reasons does so at his peril ". This includes operations for purely cosmetic reasons unless it can be truthfully shown that the defect has a harmful psychological effect and its correction will be medically beneficial. Lord Brock continues, " ritual circumcision is an even worse example " and advises the surgeon not to perform it just because he is asked. It should be done on medical grounds. This should not be interpreted that Lord Brock is opposed to the ritual practice of circumcision on religious grounds, which he considers a different matter. He appreciates the existence of a religious conscience just as there is a medical one.

4

THE NATURE OF DISEASE

DISEASE might be looked upon as a change in a tissue or organ brought about by an agent, such as a bacterium or virus, or from an anomaly or defect in its formation. The doctor is generally able to demonstrate some constant defect in the tissue, a consistent response to a particular treatment or else he can predict a likely effect on life. The hypothesis of a change in the tissue corresponds with the view of Rudolf Virchow, who, looking at disease with the eyes of a scientist, declared that it is essentially a cellular disturbance. But it is not true for those diseases in which no obvious pathological lesion can be demonstrated.[1] Perhaps John Ryle's (1936) definition of disease comes nearer to mine since he regards it as the whole consequence of the conflict between man and the noxious agencies in his environment.[2]

We assume that disease is as old as or even older than man. Animals and plants too are subject to it. There is no living species which cannot be attacked by an organism or is not liable to an anomaly in its formation. It can be appreciated how certain defects or lack of a certain enzyme are followed by the loss of function in a particular organ. Further, certain organisms can be expected to gain entrance to and multiply within a normally formed body to an enormous extent when its protective mechanisms are overcome. We know there are many people who harbour pathogenic bacteria in their throats and yet remain in excellent health. But if those organisms enter the body of another person or if, for any reason, the indi-

---

[1] Virchow, R., quoted from Rather, L. J. (1961). *Stanford med. Bull.*, **19,** 186.
[2] Ryle, J. A. (1936). *The Natural History of Disease,* 2nd ed., p. 14. London, Oxford University Press.

vidual's resistance is altered he may succumb to a serious febrile disorder, such as typhoid fever, septicaemia or pneumonia.

There is evidence that the balance of nature is maintained by one species destroying another and this in turn is kept in check by yet another *ad infinitum*. A certain environment may favour the growth of some organisms at the same time discouraging the development of others. We are told by some authorities that there tends to be less poliomyelitis in an overcrowded and less hygienic environment whereas in places with no squalor this virus may not only thrive but assume greater pathogenicity as well. In overcrowded African townships there is less poliomyelitis than in areas occupied by better off Europeans, although it can be said that the opportunity for natural immunity to develop is higher. The amoebic parasite is far more dangerous to man in the tropics than in much colder Europe where, although the parasite may be passed in the stools of some people, it rarely appears to develop invasive and pathogenic properties. Alteration of the environment therefore may render its population more susceptible to attack.

Probably the majority of bacteria and even of certain viruses are of help to man. We know how the bacterial flora in the gut assist in the manufacture of the essential vitamins which are then absorbed. We do not know in what way man, through the introduction of chemical agencies, has altered the balance of nature and we are concerned about this. There no longer exists the same number or the same species of insects. We have cleared large tracts of land and rendered them mosquito-free, but we must ask ourselves if we have not unleashed millions of organisms normally destroyed by this insect. This is a reasonable fear. Heisch (1956)[1] in Kenya has shown how plague has appeared in some parts through man changing his agricultural methods and habits. Mahaffy and his colleagues noticed that the yellow fever virus existed in the towns and was transmitted by the domestic mosquito, *Aedes aegypti,* but

[1] Heisch, R. B. (1956). *Br. med. J.,* **2,** 669.

where the towns adjoined the forest the virus was transmitted to different mosquitoes living in the tree tops and these in turn infected other cities also bordering the forest.[1] Professor Garnham reminds us that in Kenya during the last war when a few troops with the malarial parasite in their blood were brought into a region of high altitude which had before only occasionally been penetrated by man, they infected the mosquito population of this virgin area. The mosquitoes in their turn infected the rest of the troops and so severe outbreaks of malaria occurred amongst men who had not previously harboured the parasite and in an area where the disease was not normally to be expected. We know too that through the opening of new trade routes in West Africa, sleeping sickness has been introduced to many new and hitherto uninfected populations. Thus there is much evidence that man in his progressiveness has introduced disease and helped to spread it.[2]

Yet I doubt if it has been shown conclusively that destruction of an organism or an insect carrier of disease, such as the mosquito, through medical advances has been followed by an epidemic of disease. Nor can it be satisfactorily proven that interference of medical scientists with the natural environment has resulted in greater frequency of disease. For instance there has been an increase of bilharziasis where natural dams and irrigation projects have been opened in endemic regions, but medicine is hardly responsible for this. It has followed man's quest for greater agricultural gain. Similarly in England the development of asbestosis from inhalation of the fibre by those who handle it is not the result of interference by the medical profession. Doctors are aware of the dangers but they cannot prevent industrialists from harnessing the energy and products of nature for economic advantage. It is feared that with the introduction of antibiotics resistant bacteria will become so

[1] Mahaffy, A. F. (1942). *Trans. R. Soc. trop. Med. Ayq.*, **36**, 9.
[2] Garnham, P. C. C. (1965). *Theoretical Questions of Natural Foci of Diseases*, p. 267. Czechoslovak Academy of Sciences.

frequent that they may well resist all forms of known treatment and so man will be worse off than before. But as yet, on the whole, the attack on the pathogenic bacteria has met with outstanding success despite those that have become resistent to certain antibiotics.

More serious perhaps is the rise of the diseases which result from drugs supplied by the profession. For instance there seems to be a definite increase in the incidence of the connective tissue (collagen) diseases, many of which are serious and may have been caused by sulphonamides in sensitive patients. In the not uncommon disorder of acute intermittent porphyria the attack is usually precipitated when the sufferer is given barbiturates, sulphonamides or an anaesthetic containing a barbiturate. The patient, free from an attack at the time, suddenly develops this serious acute disturbance from which death may follow. There must be many iatragenic disorders or anxiety states following visits to the doctor. The patient is told he has high blood pressure, or a gastric ulcer, or some other serious disorder and this information so affects him that he becomes a hypochondriac. His mental equilibrium is disturbed by fears that have been engendered or implanted in his mind by his physician's remarks or manner. We can think of many disorders that follow the doctor's endeavours.

Medicine can also claim some credit for the increase of population in many countries of the world today. The great sanitary revolution, improved surgical techniques, better medical treatment and care of the child against infectious diseases have all helped in their own decisive way to lessen the mortality in childbirth and infancy.

The Art and Science of Medicine

With the phenomenal development of mathematics, physics, and chemistry in the 18th and 19th centuries the scientific outlook became more firmly entrenched in procedures adopted by the medical man. Moral, ethical and perhaps religious aspects of medicine began to assume a lesser role, although they still retained a place of respect and consideration in medical thought. At the close of the 19th century medical men showed some concern at the largely scientific outlook that was beginning to manifest itself in medicine. Perhaps this was the start of a great era in which European thought, led by positivists like Durkheim, saw truth only in science. Europe had moved away from the philosophical or metaphysical approach to human problems. Only the sciences mattered. But in European countries, notably France and Italy, there arose a fear of this objective, positivistic attitude. Bergson and Sorel of France, and Croce of Italy each gave the world a new spiritual uplift in thought. Has medical thought not been influenced by these men? Has the medical profession remained unmoved and accepted to the full the teachings of Richard Bright, Humphry Davy, Louis Pasteur and Lister? It seems that science has won the day and gained a firm grip on the practice of medicine. Those concerned admit that the science of medicine, the science of knowledge, with its objective approach, cannot be doubted and must be accepted. Yet we constantly hear the cry that medicine is also an art which is being lost. Doctors are becoming mere scientists or technicians without paying attention to the equally important aspect of their calling, the art, philosophy, or call it what you will, of being personal. Many are disturbed about this. Some try to define this so-called art of medicine, but I am not satisfied as to its proper meaning and its existence as something special to medicine. It is not merely the ability to handle people in difficult situations or an understanding of human beings for surely this competency is equally expected of a general in battle, a business manager in his store or the chief secretary in a government department. I see in their protest a more subtle meaning, an attempt to define the essence of medicine. Medicine does not merely involve matters originating from a disturbed function due to the absence or destruction of a cell. It is not concerned only with a physical defect. In medicine there are also disturbances which we cannot measure by a piece of scientific apparatus. Some of them are metaphysical, due to some factor far beyond the ken of men, believed by the medical expert to exist in Nature. Perhaps this unknown force, factor or whatever its nature, causes the nervous breakdown, the anxiety state, the psychosomatic disturbances, backache and joint pains. Every day in his practice the clinician tries to account for the many disorders which cannot be explained except in vague terms, such as " overwork," " overstrain," " lack of holiday," " financial worry," " going out in the cold," " having a cold bath " etc. There is a sub-conscious resistance to the scientific approach which cannot explain everything. Perhaps it is the emotional reaction of these medical men who speak of the art of medicine. Freud's hypotheses and approach to the causation of mental disease, followed by those of Jung, Adler and others, also leave us doubtful as to whether we have made true headway in this important field of medicine. I must admit that some new opening or discovery in medicine which follows the scientific approach may well show us one day that all diseases can be explained scientifically. Then philo-sophical and metaphysical argument will no longer be feasible. When this happens the need for the religious or spiritual role in disease may well fall by the way, but until that day, which is apparently still a long way off, there remains strong support for those who believe that medicine is metaphysical as well as scientific.

How does the Public View Disease?

How the general public views medicine depends on the public concerned. If a sample was selected from New York, London or Berlin, we might expect the majority of these people to postulate that disease is due to a germ that has entered the body. There it multiplies and disease follows, the particular symptoms that ensue depending on the site affected. If we chose our population sample from the centre of the Congo the answer would be entirely different. Here the con-sensus of opinion would be that disease is produced by an angered spirit or a witch; in other words it is due to some preternatural agency. This is easily explained. The African peoples regard the origin of disease as spiritual. The European on the other hand has gradually moved away from this concept, due to various sources of education over the years, although he might still accept that there is also a supernatural influence to be considered in the production of disease. In any Christian society it is difficult to know how often people pray to God for His help to overcome the illness and restore the sick one to health. Prayers for the sick are made daily in churches. It must therefore be accepted that the Christian recognises two factors that influence an illness. Not only is reliance placed on the medical man and in science but also on prayer. How much more faith is placed in medicine than in God is impossible to say as this varies from person to person. In truth the spiritual or religious connection with disease may be slight but cognisance of this must be taken, for it colours the attitude of the public to the medical man.

EPISTEMOLOGICAL VALIDITY

Which of these various types of epistemology has the greatest validity? The bulk of the authorised and " degreed " medical practitioners would claim that the answer is the scientific theory and if the various types of epistemology were tested by a selection of diseases to be cured, I have no doubt which theory would provide the greatest number of successes. It would be the scientific theory. In fact, the final validity for a medical epistemology is that it is better than any other, in cures and in the alleviation of disease. And thus, final validity must surely be awarded to the scientific theory.

However, does this mean that the other epistemologies have no validity or application in practice at all? No, I believe that some have a place in medical practice. The number of cases of disease in which the scientific theory has not helped, and one of the non-scientific types has, are many. The non-scientific practitioners often cannot explain why their method was effective, but this is of no consequence as long as the aims of medicine are upheld—to cure and alleviate disease.

The state of scientific knowledge about disease is far from perfect and will probably remain so for centuries, and while this is the case no stone can be left unturned where the patient's health is concerned, even if the non-scientific method is a thorn in the flesh of the scientific doctor.

5

THE DOCTOR

Who is the Medical Man?

A MEDICAL man should first be concerned with the recognition or diagnosis of a person's ailment and/or take a direct part in its treatment. We can argue that he must have passed a recognised state examination. A doctor is a person who has a direct concern in some way or another with the patient, be he a general practitioner or engaged in a particular speciality. As long as he is in direct contact at some stage of the illness he must be regarded as a doctor. In some instances the doctor does the whole examination, investigation and treatment on his own. In this way he may do a good deal for the patient, but in other instances he resorts to assistance from a surgeon, physician, dermatologist, psychiatrist or some other specialist who can also be regarded as a doctor. Therefore as long as there has been a personal or responsible relationship with the sick person, short or long, he can be accepted as being a doctor. Thus there may be several doctors concerned in the recovery of the patient.

It can be said with very good reason that the witchdoctor of Africa sees and treats his patients and none can dispute his belief that he too is helping them; many of his clientele too consider that they have responded to his administrations. We can argue *ad infinitum* about the witchdoctor's criterion of cure which in the eyes of Western doctors lacks scientific proof. But his claims today are perhaps no less scientific than were those of Western doctors who practised about 500 years ago in Britain, with what we should call a pseudo-scientific method of treatment. Yet the doctor of that period was accepted. Why then do we not accept the witchdoctor as a proper doctor?

He has not followed a scientific method of approach. He has not undergone a training in anatomy or physiology or followed an objective approach to the causation of disease. He does not recognise that in disease structural changes take place in the cells or tissues. He is totally unaware of the science of pathology. He has no concept of a microscopic lens. His arguments as to the cause of disease are mystical, for he says that illness and death are due to an angered spirit or to the influence of one of the patient's dead relatives. There is no positive proof that this is true. He disregards the laws of science and bases his claims on impressions; in consequence we cannot accept him as a proper medical man. The witch-doctor is required to undergo a special period of initial training —mostly spiritual—or apprenticeship with another of his calling. He sits no examinations but he is expected to have practised his art for some months or years before he is publicly acclaimed as an accepted medical man at a ritual ceremony, at which thanks are offered to the healing spirit which has served his family for generations. He keeps his knowledge to himself as a jealously guarded secret. What he learns from others in his apprenticeship or, as is more often claimed, through his special hereditary healing spirit, he does not share with his colleagues. He does not confer with them. He is not called in by other witchdoctors to help when a patient does not recover, but he has no objection to his patient leaving him and seeking another opinion. Secrecy is part of his calling for he believes that if he were to divulge his knowledge he would upset the ancestral spirit to which he owes his spiritual talent. This is the opposite of the Hippocratic doctor whose knowledge is not kept secret. Any experience he gains he is ready to make known in a medical journal. He holds regular consultations with other doctors in the presence of his patients and goes to conferences, so that all can benefit from the common fund of knowledge. This is expected of those who follow the scientific approach and seek the truth. It can be argued that members of other healing cults, like faith-healers, do not practise secretly and only consult with their own colleagues in the same way as doctors. But though the medical profession does not differ from them in these aspects it does on its Newtonian approach.

When there is no direct contact between the patient and a qualified doctor the position becomes debatable. For instance take a pathologist sitting in his office merely signing a laboratory form that a blood count has been carried out on the patient. Can we call him a true doctor? Are we to include the medical officer of health, who, when employed in a purely administrative capacity, is not in contact with any patient? Strictly speaking he is not a doctor but a specialist official. It would not be correct to regard the chief medical officer of health who never sees patients as a doctor. He may have practised medicine once, but the moment he gives up the contact and responsibility of his patients he moves into another field. This does not mean that his specialist professional skill is not worthy of the highest regard. Indeed his skill, training and knowledge are often far greater than those of the medical practitioner and his contributions may even exceed those of the practising clinician. Nevertheless it can be said that he is not a doctor in the true sense of the word. He neither sees, diagnoses nor treats a patient any more than does the technician in the laboratory or the radiographer who takes a plate of an enlarged heart or the ambulance driver who rushes the sick man into hospital. All play their parts and all are essential. In some the skill and training are above those of the doctor, in others the level is lower. No one denies that the ambulance driver or the first-aid attendant at a football match plays an important part; so does the policeman who is called to see a person knocked down in the street. Take a person practising medicine by rendering important first-aid until the patient can be brought into hospital, could he not be said to be a medical man since he has treated an injured person and is following a recognised procedure? However, as he has not passed the required examination he cannot be considered a doctor. Thus

4

to be a true doctor there are two requirements. The first is that he must pass the set examination and the second that he must assume some degree of personal responsibility or contact with the sick person.

The Good Doctor

The good doctor must be one who believes in and follows the aims of medicine. Therefore he is the person who, when called upon, helps any individual to restore or maintain his health or that of the community by preventing the start of an illness. But unorthodox practitioners, such as the spiritualist or faithhealer, may point out that this is their object as well. However if a person wishes to practise as a doctor he has to complete the curriculum of study in the various subjects laid down in an accepted institution of learning and after passing its examination he is required to register with the recognised medical body in the particular country where he proposes to practice. The study of medicine is scientific. It has certain well-defined principles which must be followed in order to fulfil the aim of medicine according to its definition.

The basic principles which determine what is a good doctor do not change. Yet the impression exists that men in contemporary practice are better doctors than their predecessors. It is true that the present day practitioner is armed with far more technical knowledge—radioactive isotopes, enzymes, image itensifiers and other scientific aids which help in the recognition of disease. Yet none of the great doctors like William Harvey, Joseph Lister and Patrick Manson had any of these facilities. None can say that they were less useful in their calling as doctors than those of today. These men and others only one or two generations ago were imbued with the same approach we have now. They studied the patient's history, then examined him and tested the urine. Admittedly with the use of the microscope in clinical medicine, the newer advances in chemistry and the discovery of the roentgen rays, the whole face of medicine has altered. Every succeeding generation will find that its doctors are better equipped than those who have just preceded them.

It must be confessed that the more facilities there are at the disposal of the clinician the more certain and less open to error will be his diagnosis. A doctor of 100 years ago would probably have diagnosed diabetes purely on the presence of sugar in the urine and so would have missed a number of diabetics because he could not carry out a blood sugar test in order to discover those with a high renal threshold. The doctor today can detect the diabetic patient more accurately. He can also claim that he saves more lives. Thus he is more positively of value to society than his colleagues who practised centuries back and therefore it would be reasonable to say that he is a better doctor in this aspect of his work. For all that, the fact must be faced that the doctor of the nineteenth century was a much respected man, held in high regard by his patients. His advice, help and encouragement were sought far and wide. With his black bag and his bottle of coloured medicine he was still very welcome in the homes of the sick. No doubt he could recognise when a patient was suffering from lobar pneumonia. He possibly knew more about the natural history of disease. But his failure to cure many diseases was more frequent as compared with the results achieved today. We can find numerous examples of beloved doctors who practised a hundred years ago and were highly respected by the people for their skill in handling ailments. Dr Henry Bickersteth, M.D., F.R.C.S., who came from Britain, was a hospital surgeon in the Somerset Hospital at Cape Town. He practised there for a good number of years and when he died in 1872 the whole city went into mourning and a tablet in his memory was erected in St. George's Cathedral of that city. What could Bickersteth have done as a surgeon in 1870 when we take into consideration the wonderful strides in the science of surgery since his day, when the impact of Lister's antiseptic methods had not yet reached this part of the world? Bickersteth was as much loved by the people of Cape Town as any surgeon there today where many outstanding surgeons are in practice. Goodness and quality are relative.

The quality of a doctor depends on his acceptance of the principle that his main function is to help and on his desire to aid anyone in poor health. As long as he is interested in the welfare of the sick and employs the best remedial measures possible for that purpose and shows that he is to be trusted, he will not lack many friends and supporters—people who turn to him in times of sickness. He will be accepted and appreciated by his fellow men. A recovery is likely to be attributed to the wise choice of his medicine and as most ill-nessess end happily with recovery, the doctor's chances of a favourable outcome are good. Further by trial and error over centuries many useful empirical remedies have come into use. Even if the doctor of long ago had none of the wonder drugs of today, by careful choice of the mixtures, which had bene-ficial pharmacological effects, the chances of recovery were greatly improved. Thus, whilst he had few specific remedies for disease, yet in the early stages, where, for instance, a painful and distressing cough was troublesome, a sedative cough mixture was rational treatment. Even nowadays a loss— through no fault of the doctor—very often wins the gratitude of the family for his efforts to assist to the last. He comes to be trusted and loved in spite of the death of the patient. Many close relationships are set up at the time of a family crisis when the patient's struggle for survival is acute and desperate. During these days or weeks the family may come to remember the doctor with gratitude.

The doctor is concerned with the individual and his com-plaint. In this role he can never be replaced. During sickness family ties become stronger, more real and a rallying point for those connected, who, in their turn feel and even suffer with the sick one. Therefore in order to handle the patient's complaints effectively the doctor must at the same time be able to cope with the feelings of the family. He is no longer concerned merely with the patient and his future, but is immediately bound up with the welfare of the entire group. He must be able to handle them sensibly and sympathetically. Indeed on occasions like this, tense with the threat of death, the ability of the doctor comes to the fore. He is now not so much the scientist as the organiser or administrator who is able to handle those who are distressed at the impending or possible loss of their dear one. At such a time he can no longer be the exact scientist only but has also to remember that the individual's sickness is the focal point for all those concerned.

It is the effort that the doctor puts into a case that counts. Even though a doctor nowadays is able to treat effectively a person stricken with lobar pneumonia or malaria, the patient and his immediate family often take the treatment as a matter of course. He is pleased he is better but sees no special reason to be impressed with the doctor. All that was needed was done with pills. Perhaps the patient is more grateful to the antibiotics than to the doctor. On the whole in the days when there were no antibiotics, no ambulances or nursing homes, the doctor was more in the picture, taking his stand by the patient and almost shared his battle. The close liaison and dependence of the patient on the doctor has become less and less with the advance of scientific treatment.

I have been trying to convey that there has always been a high place for the doctor through the many centuries when he was asked to cope with the anxieties of man. No matter what his standard of knowledge and scientific qualifications were or how they compared from one century to the next, he had to play the role of a comforter to the sick individual. No matter how limited his knowledge might have been, he was still a much sought-after person, even when much of what he did was largely unscientific. Why for so long has there been a place for the doctor in the treatment of disease? It was mostly because he treated the patient and not only the disease. Thus if the present day doctor with the added technical knowledge at his disposal, remembers not to lose touch with his patient in his endeavour to treat the disease, he will be a good doctor.

The Doctor's Virtues

Almost every virtue has been claimed as necessary for the good doctor. About 1400 schoolmasters in Britain were asked what qualities they considered a boy should possess if he intended to take up medicine. Amongst the more important ones stressed were loyalty, perseverance, poise, conscientiousness, sympathy, patience, compassion, gentleness and imagination.[1]

For centuries qualities necessary for the good doctor have been elaborated. The great Paracelsus spoke of two kinds of physicians, those who worked for love and those who worked for their own profit. They were both known by their works; the true and just physician, he claimed, was recognised by his unfailing love for his neighbour, whereas the unjust ones were known by their transgressions, for they were to be likened to ravenous wolves since all they wanted was to increase their profit and heeded not the commandment of love. Paracelsus urged that since the physician was created by God and not by man he should act in good faith and without lying.

When doctors themselves write on the requirements of the good doctor, they expect almost every virtue in him. Gilchrist (1963)[2] says that he must be welcome in society as well as being a man of good education and good manners.

Robert Louis Stevenson was also particular about the sort of doctor he liked. This is how he described him in the " Dedication " of his collection of poems " Underwoods."

" There are men and classes of men that stand above the common herd; the soldier, the sailor, and the shepherd not unfrequently; the artist rarely; rarelier still, the clergyman, the physician almost as a rule. He is the flower (such as it is) of our civilisation; and when that stage of man is done with, and only remembered to be marvelled at in history, he will be thought to have shared as little as any in the defects of the

---

[1] British Medical Association (1962). B.M.A. Publications. *Becoming a Doctor: A Guide to careers in Medicine,* p. 16. London.
[2] Gilchrist, A. R. (1963). *Lancet,* **2,** 1.

period, and most notably exhibited the virtues of the race. Generosity he has, such as is possible to those who practise an art, never to those who drive a trade; discretion, tested by a hundred secrets; tact, tried in a thousand embarrassments; and, what are more important, Heraclean cheerfulness and courage. So it is that he brings air and cheer into the sickroom, and often enough, though not so often as he wishes, brings healing."[1]

A fairly popular virtue stressed by other doctors is the understanding heart. What is meant by this? The philosopher Martin Buber says in his criticism of contemporary man that he tends to regard the other person as an " it " rather than " thou " and that the " I-thou " relationship of respect is hardly ever observed today. Curran (1964),[2] a minister of religion (in the United States of America) appeals for the understanding doctor who displays a consideration and regard for his patient. Steiger (1963)[3] too demands " the understanding doctor who is able to appreciate the subjective feelings of his patient." But he warns against thinking that all that is required from the understanding doctor is love or sympathy. He should rather be aware of and understand the particular situation in which he finds the patient. He should be able to feel with him. Steiger claims that patients need this contact and that even with a limited amount of scientific background healing can take place in such an atmosphere.

But sympathy in a doctor can be overdone. Blumgart (1964)[4] warns against it. He says it is doubtful if the doctor should enter into the feelings of the patient and become similarly affected. Sympathy should refer to an affinity between doctor and patient so that the former understands and appreciates

[1] The works of Robert Louis Stevenson. Swanston Edition, 1912. Vol. 14, p. 63. Chatto & Windus, London.
[2] Curran, C. A. (1964). *J. Am. med. Ass.,* **188,** 140.
[3] Steiger, W. A. (1963). *J. med. Educ.,* **38,** 768.
[4] Blumgart, H. L. (1964). *New Engl. J. Med.,* **270,** 449.

what affects the latter and so is able to move with him in his difficulties.

Other doctors advocate that the practitioner should be able to see his own frailties, to laugh at them, forgive himself and others—in other words he should have a sense of humour. Stevens (1964)[1] links humility with a sense of humour for when these two qualities are combined the doctor is unlikely to become self important and so has a truer perception of what he is and of the public. Paracelsus says much the same—no doctor should be arrogant—and Marti-Ibanez (1963)[2] considers the hall-mark of a physician, like that of any man, is humility.

Tarlov (1964)[3] warns that a doctor should never " bluff ", by which he means that he should not pretend to have knowledge which he does not possess. It is essential for him to pursue the truth. His best method to discover what the patient is suffering from is the Hippocratic approach which has already been described and once having found out the truth he must treat his patient along those lines. At this stage the doctor may find himself in a dilemma. There are some to whom he can tell the truth, but there are others who, on being told the true nature of their complaints, may become so disturbed that they lose all hope and will to live. There are a few doctors who maintain that whatever his reaction the patient must be told the exact nature of his illness so he can come to terms with his fate. Whether he believes the patient must be told or not, he must certainly inform some responsible member of the family or the person's guardian of the truth. Such a discussion may help to decide whether or not it is better to tell the patient what is the matter with him. Therefore a doctor should not feel dishonest if he withholds the information from the patient provided a responsible member of the family knows and considers it in the patient's interest not to tell him.

[1] Stevens, H. (1964). *J. Am. med. Ass.*, **190**, 1114.
[2] Marti-Ibanez, F. (1963). *Ariel*: *Essay on the Arts and the History and Philosophy of Medicine*. MD Publications Inc., New York.
[3] Tarlov, I. M. (1964). *N.Y. St. J. Med.*, **64**, 1769.

What should be the doctor's attitude towards telling his patient the true nature of the drug he is prescribing for him or the risks involved in an operation he has advised? The problem is a complicated one. Firstly, the doctor should avoid if possible frightening the patient or his family lest he refuse the treatment and so endanger his life. Further, patients with a particular psychological make-up may develop an anxiety state if told about such risks. So much depends on how he puts the matter to the patient for an ill-advised warning or badly chosen words may rouse all kinds of fears. An adverse reaction may follow a penicillin injection, a sulpha drug or even a dose of aspirin. Therefore the doctor should weigh up the chances of anything going amiss since every patient should realise that there is just a small risk in taking any drug and that an unexpected reaction may follow an anaesthetic. The position is easier in the case of an operation as a written consent has to be obtained beforehand and therefore before the anaesthetic is administered. But is the doctor to warn his patient every time he prescribes aspirin or phenobarbitone as the risk is so slight? On the other hand, with a drug that has specific harmful effects on a vital part of the body the doctor should explain to the patient that there are certain risks attached to it, but that they are most unlikely if care is taken with regard to its correct indication and dosage and the pre-cautions outlined followed. This should be remembered with drugs like emetine, antimony, arsenic or any new drug of which he has had little experience himself but knows that its pharmacological tests have been considered favourable. When the risk is relatively slight but cannot be altogether dismissed the doctor should protect his patient and himself by carrying out beforehand the recognised procedures, such as sensitivity tests, and enquire into allergic reactions of the patient to certain drugs, pointing out at the same time that they may produce some reactions but that he himself has very rarely met them. When performing a procedure like a lumbar puncture it is wise for the doctor to cover himself by telling the patient that it might cause a little headache or discomfort but there is no real risk of this. Selecting the right details and choosing his words carefully, depending on the mental make-up of the patient, is very important so as not to alarm him. Clearly the more risky the procedure, the more dangerous the drug, the more necessary it is to tell the patient and those concerned about it. Thus if amphoterecin B is being used the patient should be informed about its dangers, but in such a case he would be so seriously ill that he and his family would realise that such a heroic measure has to be used.

Sir Robert Aitken[1] calls for a better relationship between doctor and patient and even between nurse and patient, since the professional tends to become too technical, academic and impersonal. Some doctors, he says, should be more approachable and less like inaccessible gods. He even pleads that the doctor himself should take a careful history of the patient on every occasion since a medical interview has an influence on the sick person and this is in itself a form of psychological therapy. He is opposed to any attempt to reduce the clinical history to a standardised questionnaire. The consultation must be held in a private place with the doctor face to face with the patient. The medical history thus gained through personal contact is the constant golden thread of medicine.

But all these qualities in a person do not necessarily make him a good doctor. A doctor with good manners, sympathy and a pleasant personality has a good start, but he needs something more. I have known many who lack one or more of these virtues. Some could be rude, lose their tempers and treat their patients shabbily, yet they managed to keep their practices because they knew their work, were capable and could be relied upon in any emergency to do their best for those who put their trust in them. Their patients could have absolute confidence in them. What matters most is that a good doctor should understand the aims of medicine. He must know and pursue the truth. If unfortunately he has a quick temper or is

[1] Aitken, R. (1964). *Australas. Ann. Med.* **13,** 279.

ill-mannered that does not make him a poor doctor. It is well to remember that there is always the exception to every rule.

Self Deception

Even a body of men like the medical profession, which has always prided itself on its honesty, can practise self deception. For centuries it treated acute malaria by venesection, believing that the evil cause of the ague could be removed from the body. This appears a rational argument if it were believed as it was at that time, that the fever was caused by inhaling noxious vapour. The existence of a parasite in the blood which invaded the blood stream from the liver was unknown. So blood was removed making the patient more anaemic and thus adding to his distress. No doctor today would attempt such a practice. In fact in acute malaria it is much more likely that a severely ill person will need a blood transfusion. How many men lost their lives through venesection will never be known, yet doctors continued this procedure for centuries, believing they were pursuing a useful treatment. They shut their eyes to its effect on their patients. When the ill-fated ship the " Congo " entered the Congo River in 1817 the surgeon bled the men with fever. Again when the great Niger Expedition ascended the Niger River in 1840 the surgeons on most of the ships bled their men with frightful results. Yet none questioned the method of treatment. If only the profession had compared results in those bled with those not bled the answer would have been so different.

There was a similar resistance on the part of the medical profession to Lister's new antiseptic techniques. We ask why were the learned and leading surgeons so opposed to it when the results of their operations were so frightful and the losses so heavy. Yet for years they continued to oppose Lister in spite of his publications that revealed such convincing figures. They had shut their minds to the truth and deceived themselves.

In everyday practice no matter what our special field, we must always remember to keep an open mind, one which is flexible and not resistant to new ideas or suggestions. At times a new concept is irritating and our reaction is to reject it. The temptation arises to dismiss a claim out of hand. Yet if the results of a treatment are unsatisfactory, there is always reason to expect a better approach. We might expect that with age and experience the older doctor is ready to accept new advances, but this is by no means always the case. Indeed with increasing age it is more difficult for a doctor to recognise new ideas. Although it is important to know the source of the information or the claim, its author and centre of research, we should guard against prejudices and not dismiss it if it stems from places which may not have such great standing in academic circles. Whilst as a rule, better work is expected from the great universities, not infrequently the most outstanding advances come from places whence they are least expected.

The Doctor : His Service to his Public or to his Profession

How do we assess a doctor's work? If this could be done satisfactorily it would be a useful index of his services to the sick. In order to determine how to assess his value we might begin by considering exactly what he does in his daily work and what he is trying to achieve for himself.

If we look at the medical profession, we notice that there are broadly speaking two kinds of doctors. There is the one who directs his energies towards rendering useful service to man through the scientific approach. This leads him to a better understanding of disease and its prevention. He works mostly with his colleagues and publishes his findings in medical journals. His urge is to acquire more knowledge through working for higher diplomas and special degrees and to become an acknowledged authority on disease. He is more attracted to academic life. The public are his patients to whom he is generally respectful, sympathetic and even kind, but they are of secondary consideration to his life's ambition. He works for an ideal and the pleasure of achievement that his scientific contributions bring him and if honours come his way through recognition by his colleagues, their colleges or other learned bodies he is more than happy to accept them. Such men may hope to become president of one of the medical colleges or serve in one of the medical associations through which they may find an outlet for their special interests. The field therefore is very wide, stretching from pure science to medical politics.

The second type of doctor serves the sick who are his main interest. This doctor is not so much the pure scientist or academician who learns or gains his knowledge by experience. He prefers to learn from the medical scientists and then apply what he has gleaned. He is happiest when concerned with the problems and welfare of his patients and their families. He is basically the doctor of the individual or the family unit. Most of all he wants to see each of them through their illnesses. He is the family friend and standby in all sorts of crises. This type of doctor is found not only amongst general practitioners although it would be true to say that the great majority of them belong to this category. But in this group too can be included interns in hospitals, specialists, physicians and surgeons who also serve the public with similar objectives. They are well known to the public with whom they are on much more intimate terms than are the medical scientists. The public thinks highly of them and is attached to them. On the other hand, the public understands very little of what the medical scientist is striving for except what it learns from the press. Perhaps Bernard Shaw[1] failed to understand the medical profession when he wrote in his *The Doctor's Dilemma* that the rank and file of doctors were no more men of science than baboons. He did not realise that to the medical practitioner doctoring was an " art " and not only a science.

Nothing attracts the public so much as the idea of sacrifice by a doctor in the interests of his fellow men. Personal sacrifice on its behalf appeals more than scientific discoveries, which, although impressive, are impersonal and distant. There is no doubt that the public is grateful to Dr. Salk and Dr. Sabin

[1] Shaw, B. (1946). *The Doctor's Dilemma*. Penguin Books, London.

for their contributions on the poliomyelitis vaccine. On the other hand, Dr. Albert Schweitzer has achieved great fame because of his life of service alone. Here was a doctor with a promising career ahead of him in the musical and theological world, who gave up all that Europe had to offer and chose to work instead in the heat of tropical Africa where he cared for lepers and others for the rest of his days. For money to run his hospital at Lambarene he organised concerts in Europe. The heart of the world was touched by such great personal sacrifice, by the man who gave up everything for the sake of the sick.

Equally great in the public mind was Dr. David Livingstone. In his efforts to find a healthy mission station he made many geographical discoveries. He was mainly a Christian missionary but when he died near the swamps of Lake Bangweulu the English world proclaimed him a national hero and he was buried with honours in Westminster Abbey. The world was not so much taken with his discovery of the so-called " Livingstone pill " for malaria or impressed because he was the first to recognise the tick as the transmitting agent of relapsing fever but rather by the supreme sacrifice he made for humanity. But there are many other Schweitzers and Livingstones. Many of them, although they served the cause of Christianity, were first and foremost medical men. There were so many medical missionaries who went to Asia and Africa that it is difficult to mention them all. Many seem to have been forgotten and only a few of their fine names survive. Some left their mark on the public mind and are still gratefully remembered for their services. One such man was William Affleck Scott who worked in 1890 at the Blantyre mission in Malawi and never ceased helping the sick. In those days when there was no proper transport and the roads were treacherous the sick had to be carried into Blantyre on litters (machilas). Once Dr. Scott had to travel 40 miles to see a sick African in the rainy season. He was not well at the time and so went out to him in a machila. There he decided that the sick man needed to be brought in to Blantyre so he gave the patient his machila and walked by his side on the return journey. As there was no hospital he often treated his patients in his own home and performed operations in his kitchen. As he was doubly qualified, in order to retain his identity as a doctor and not a minister, he wore ordinary clothes. He died whilst still a comparatively young man. The people of Blantyre mourned his passing and remembered him suitably with a plaque to his memory in the mission church. But the public did not remember its fine medical missionaries only. There are hundreds of instances of doctors who were honoured for the services they gave. For example, there was a Dr. Donaldson who practised for many years in the little Rhodesian town of Selukwe, a small mining village with a few farms around it. During the 1918 flu epidemic his unceasing efforts for the many sick aroused the admiration of the public and when he died some years later they named their maternity home after him.

Perhaps the best testimonial for a doctor is the recognition he receives from both the public and the medical profession. This does happen, for the good doctor who practises wisely will be able to satisfy his patients and win their approval and at the same time by his accurate diagnoses, approach and procedures receive acknowledgment of his value by the medical world. The best qualified doctor is the one who is accepted as worthwhile by both his patients and his colleagues.

Reputation

The doctor cannot simply think only of himself and his own affairs for he is not quite like a business man who is concerned only with his business and his financial reward. The business man derives pleasure from the growth and development of his project. It is true he may even be able to perceive good that he is doing for mankind. But a doctor is different. He is concerned not so much with monetary gain as with the welfare of his patients. How often have I heard at the conclusion of any debate on a medical argument, " It is the patient who counts in the long run", " the patient is always right " or " the patient comes first ". The doctor has to forego his own interests for those of his patients.

The doctor is in a different category to most other people because, although he earns his living from his work, his work goes far beyond this. Much of his life is devoted to healing the sick. Therefore his first consideration should be for the patient and not for his own reputation. Even if he never reaches the top of the medical tree he has given his best to his patients and has rendered as fine a service as anyone who has been fortunate enough to become famous in medicine.

The fear is continually voiced that a scientific training tends to make a person cold and lacking in compassion and affection. Appeals often go forth to students and doctors not to forget the philosophical or human aspect of their work, kindness of heart and humility in order to prevent themselves from becoming cold scientists (Tarlov, 1964).[1]

It is even said that the cold atmosphere of the scientific doctor, as opposed to the cordial attitude of friendly assurance which should exist between the doctor and his patient, has swung public opinion against the medical man (Bradford, 1963).[2] Gilchrist (1963)[3] also differentiates between the cool, calculating, critical and detached science of medicine and the art of medicine which implies the general management of the patient with human understanding. Felix Marti-Ibanez (1963)[4] would like the doctor to be both a scientist and a human being who displays a kind heart and acts as an intermediary between the patient and God.

But there is no real proof that the scientist is cold or even cool. It is clear to a medical educationalist, such as Ellis, that the modern doctor must be well indoctrinated in the newer techniques of science. He must think more and more scientifically and because science demands integrity, this in itself

[1] Tarlov, I. M. (1964). *N.Y. St. J. Med.,* **64,** 1769.
[2] Bradford, C. H. (1963). *New Engl. J. Med.,* **268,** 1147.
[3] Gilchrist, A. R. (1963). *Lancet,* **2,** 1.
[4] Marti-Ibanez, F. (1963). *Ariel.* MD Publications Inc., New York.

will be appreciated by the patient and serve to establish trust between him and the doctor (Ellis, 1964).[1]

And how can the doctor develop a scientific mind? In answer to this question Gilchrist recommends the Baconian advice : " . . . the desire to seek, the patience to doubt, the fondness to meditate, the slowness to assert, the readiness to reconsider, the carefulness to dispose and set in order . . . and to hate every kind of imposture."

" Nor Lose the Common Touch "

A doctor's work must bring him into contact with all classes of society. He is a healer of people and therefore has to know all men whatever their walk in life. Their behaviour and reactions to disease are his concern and interest. He can learn something from every level of society. Indeed certain diseases appear more commonly in one group than another. I need not elaborate on this. Disease brings suffering and therefore we have to discover the cause of the patient's distress in order to institute treatment. He treats the poor and the rich, the able and the less able. He shares his experience with all human beings. His love for men is such that he likes them as men and does not discriminate. As William Blake wrote, everything which lives is holy.

Is the rich man entitled to a better service than a poor man or one less fortunate? It may be argued that because a man is poor and therefore more mouths are dependent on his recovery he is more deserving of specialist skill than the rich man who has probably made good provision for his family. On the other hand, the rich man may be of more vital concern to the state, or he may be the manager of an essential industry. It should not matter whether the man is rich or poor, important or not ; the principle is that all should receive equal care and attention. The poor are not entitled to more than the rich, nor the rich to more than the poor ; both deserve the same.

[1] Ellis, J. R. (1964). J. med. Educ., 39, 7.

It can be said that because the rich man has earned and saved more money he should, if he can afford it, see any doctor he wishes to consult. Further, it may so happen that he can avail himself of those costly diagnostic and therapeutic procedures which the poor man cannot afford. This is no fault of the doctor. The rich man is often at an advantage compared to the less-well-off man or one living far from centres where such facilities are available. This is understandable. But it is especially important for the doctor to remember that where the facilities are available no difference should be made between the patients who receive these aids. They should be equally available to all and the state service should not be regarded as intended only for the poor. It is there as much for the better-off and even for the millionaire if he wishes to avail himself of the facilities offered by the State. No criticism should be made if he uses them. He has contributed his share to the medical benefits of the land. The doctor may thus often find himself in a difficult position but he can do no better than serve all alike with realism and understanding.

We are aware of what many of the great clinicians of Britain achieved before the National Health Act was introduced. Many of them gave their services freely and voluntarily to the people and spent many hours attending the poor. They served in the institutions in which many of them made their reputations and showed deep affection and loyalty for their hospitals. At the same time they served the better-off patients. They did not lose the common touch.

In Britain today the face of medical practice has changed and the honorary physician and surgeon we once knew have virtually disappeared. But the social strata remain and the doctor must show the same interest in every human being. The practitioner who sees only a rich clientele is no better than the one who is content with the poorer classes. He should not make it his ambition to seek only those in more fortunate circumstances.

Before the days of the National Health Service in Britain we often heard it said that only the poor and the rich could receive adequate treatment whilst those of the middle class were the sufferers. The poor could receive free admission to voluntary hospitals and the rich could afford heavy fees. The large middle class—an important section of the public—must thus have been denied the best and more highly skilled services. This again was no more the doctor's fault than is the high incidence of a social disease. Such matters are beyond his control. But then the British Government wisely intervened and provided a service from which all could benefit. It is not a complete state service but it has provided good facilities for all classes.

No matter what his political views a doctor must be able to treat the sick whatever their political beliefs. This is not very easy always. He may well find he is tending patients with all kinds of views. It is right that he should treat all alike with the same care, kindness and attention. I am certain the patients realise this and make allowances for his not holding the same views as them. The doctor need not feel uncomfortable if he is a socialist and his patient a fascist. He has been chosen as the doctor because his patient trusts him. This is the vital point— the selection of a doctor is a matter of trust. The patient realises only too well that a man's character is what matters not his political or religious feelings. Many Christians choose a Jewish doctor and vice versa. The doctor/patient relationship is very deep and real. It is the basis of human intercourse—an understanding between human beings. Trust, confidence, inward liking and realism are qualities far deeper than the political or religious pronouncements of any individual.

With the development of modern very costly techniques, the doctor in charge of such a unit is placed in a difficult position for selecting the relatively few cases that can be treated. This is particularly evident in Britain, for instance, in a chronic haemodialysis unit, as the doctor may have to choose one out of ten applicants to receive this very specialised therapy. He may feel that for every person he treats, he is condemning to death the other nine, who are unable to receive this treatment. We know that more patients treated in this way survive for longer than five years than do patients with other incurable diseases. But the cost of this treatment is prohibitive to almost all, except a very few, since it requires an initial outlay of £400 as well as a maintenance cost of £1,000 a year for the patient to survive. Therefore people have to turn to the State or the National Health Service for help, since it is said that this service should provide the essential medical care for the several thousand cases which may require it. Since the State can only afford to provide this facility for about 10 per cent. of all cases needing it, the renal specialist is faced with the ethical problem of selecting cases of intermittent dialysis. What criteria should he adopt in selecting them? No doubt he takes into consideration the age of the patient, the cause of renal failure, the condition of the heart etc. But in addition social factors and influences are bound to intrude. Such matters as the ability of the patient to continue in regular and suitable employment, the marital state of the individual and the number of children dependent on the husband or wife. With all things equal as regards the renal disorder how does a doctor decide on grounds of priority? Should the treatment be given to a leading citizen of importance to the country or to a poor man who nevertheless has many responsibilities of his own? How is he to decree that one life is more valuable than another? Perhaps these social factors could best be determined by a lay committee and their recommendation be passed on to the renal specialist in charge of the unit to help him in his final decision. I cannot conceive that this problem is simply one of medical ethics. The issues go far beyond pure medicine. Doctors practising in emergent countries know that many lives are lost each year through lack of facilities, shortage of funds and want of specialist medical personnel. Such problems should not weigh too heavily on our medical conscience. We doctors should not feel responsible for matters beyond our control. We must recommend the best treatment available and after informing the patient of all the facts relating to such procedures and the difficulty of obtaining them refer him to a place where they are performed. Once he enters the hands of the renal specialist his general practitioner can do no more and the specialist too can only do the best possible under the circumstances. Even if he cannot give every patient the treatment he considers most suitable he has not acted contrary to the aims of medicine.[1, 2]

Who Should take up Medicine?

Who should take up medicine? The answer to this question is closely related to what the patient looks for when he chooses his doctor. The aim of the doctor is to help the sick and much thought has gone into trying to determine who is likely to make the best doctor by fulfilling this aim. There is hardly a virtue in man which has not been suggested as essential in the make up of a doctor. Some say he should be kind for if he is he will be understanding and show greater sympathy and appreciation of the situation in which the sick man finds himself. This quality is greatly favoured by the non-medical world. The need for kindness applies equally to any calling in life and no greater merit should be placed on the doctor's ability to recognise and thus cure physical disease. It is important for him to arrive at the diagnosis that explains the patient's illness. To carry this argument still further the ability to recognise and tend a patient requires a good intellect, a mental capacity of high quality not necessarily brilliant but one with good powers of weighing up the evidence, discarding unnecessary information and so coming to the right conclusion. But mental capacity is not the sole quality for everyone knows of people possessed of good brains, who are capable and have good memories yet do not necessarily pursue the truth. Many

[1] *Ethics in Medical Progress* (1966). Ciba Foundation Symposium. Edited by Wolstenholme, G. E. W. & O'Connor, M. Churchill, London.
[2] Nabarro, J. N. D., Parsons, F. M., Shackman, R. & Wilson, M. A. (1967). *Br. med. J.*, **1**, 622.

people claim that cleverness is the hallmark of a good doctor. They urge too that he must seek the truth and follow the positivist method on which true medicine is based. I believe the educationalist can detect the clever student who is able to pass examinations well. Such a person will generally be accepted to study medicine but his acceptance is based largely, although not entirely, on his examination results and this requirement comes first and is considered all-important. The ability to pursue the truth cannot be judged on examination results. It is a hidden quality and consequently many good applicants must have been refused entry to medicine through our inability to discover this. I must admit this is no one's fault. We simply do not know how to pick out this quality with any consistency at an interview.

An important attribute in a doctor, indeed in almost any profession, is the ability to work hard, not only for short periods but for day after day, month after month. This ability will certainly be of the greatest value to both patient and doctor, but once again it is difficult to know whether a youth of 18 years or so possesses it. It is a difficult virtue to assess even though a young person may show signs of it at school. The difficulty is that this ability frequently becomes evident only later in his life, often some time after qualification.

There seems to be some evidence, though rather vague, that if a child displays special interest in natural life he is likely to make a good doctor. He may enjoy wandering into the countryside collecting and dissecting insects. This interest is noted by his elders who frequently take it to denote that he should make a good doctor. David Livingstone in his early years went out gathering and studying plants and Joseph Lister too was observed to spend many hours of his youth in the countryside of Essex studying its natural life. Both these men became outstanding figures in the medical world although David Livingstone's qualities were not felt in medicine itself.

Personally I am sceptical of this alleged association between botany, animal life and medicine. I know many good medical men who never showed this interest. It is true that a child who is fond of plants or of animals has an interest in natural life. However in medicine it is not so much an interest in natural life that is required but a love for the human being. This is a real quality in a doctor, the capacity to like and respect people and one which makes him. He understands and respects the inconsistencies of man, his vicissitudes and vices, his foolishness, jealousies, heartbreaks, loves and passions, good and bad. With this attribute he is able to gain knowledge and keep in trust what he must. He knows that the brain differs from person to person, from family to family, from class to class. Yet these differences do not turn him away from people. He is attracted by this diversity of outlook and behaviour. He has come to terms with man's inconsistencies. This is the man who is wanted in the profession. The degree of kindness he possesses, good manners, the way he dresses and his outside cover are not essential qualities in his make-up. It is his love for man that matters. He wants to be with people and to help them in their troubles. This he feels is his devotion, his calling. If we could devise a method by which to discover this quality in the young we shall go a long way towards making the medical profession an even greater and more noble one than it is.

Provided he is blessed with good intelligence—an ability to grasp facts and a good memory his interest in human beings is the quality that counts more than any other single factor. If he likes and respects all mankind, rich and poor, high and low, mean and generous, he is an understanding man.

There is no single reason why a person should want to be a doctor. The obvious one is to help the sick and handicapped but this probably only applies to a rather unknown proportion of those who take up medicine. Even if an individual gives some other reason for wishing to enter the medical profession we must concede that his underlying motive is to help those in need of medical treatment. I have always been interested in the frequency with which sons and daughters of doctors enter the profession. Their choice of a medical career may be an inherent desire to follow in the footsteps of a person they admire. Further the child, as he grows up, becomes familiar with the daily routine of his father and this may provide him with a sense of confidence as he knows what is expected of a medical man. Whether the sons of doctors make better practitioners for this or other reasons we do not know for certain as it is difficult to compare different groups of doctors in actual practice.

Presumably a large number of people enter the profession as it offers an assured and satisfactory livelihood. On the whole doctors do well and are relatively more independent than those in other professions. An unknown number qualify with the object of doing well financially. But nowadays with the greater control of doctors in many European countries especially this unlimited scope has been greatly curbed and thus it would be true to say that purely material reasons for entering the profession have lessened.

We can think of other reasons for becoming doctors. It can be argued that a medical degree gives its holder a sense of power over the lives of others. A surgeon or physician can save a man from death and this realisation may have motivated some to take up this calling. Besides in the minds of many people medicine is linked with something noble and as a consequence the recruit feels he is joining a profession which has a respected status in society.

Undoubtedly there are those who are drawn to medicine by a desire to help humanity. Perhaps the missionary doctor falls into this category. Many devout Christians take up medicine with the belief that healing and prayer are in the hands of God and that they can best serve mankind by following both. David Livingstone and Albert Schweitzer are good examples, but we meet such men in other religions too. For instance the witchdoctor of Africa, although not accepted by us as a doctor, is also both a healer and a minister.

6

THE DOCTOR AND THE PUBLIC

The Doctor Alone Does not Conduct the Whole Practice of Medicine

" ON THE 14th January, 1716, four men met at St. Dunstan's Coffee House in Fleet Street. This momentous meeting led to the foundation of Westminster Hospital and later, under strange and peculiar circumstances, to the foundation of St. George's Hospital also. The four men were: Henry Hoare, banker; Robert Witham, vintner; William Wogan, writer; and the Reverend Patrick Coburn."[1] At this time there were only two other hospitals in London. No one can deny the tremendous benefit this hospital has been to London and to medicine. Yet it is noticeable that not a single doctor was present at the meeting on 14th January, 1716, when the project was launched. Doctors have the unfortunate attitude of believing that medicine begins and ends with them, that all healing and any success belongs to them alone and that few others play a significant role in medical affairs.

Some years ago I remember discussing with a medical friend how surprising it was that doctors seldom gave to or supported medical projects to help the sick and in a way themselves. They put relatively little effort into committee work or collecting funds for hospitals, preferring to confine themselves to treating the sick in them. They seem to feel that they need not make any such sacrifices, that the institutions to be erected are for their benefit and then in turn they will be helping the public. There are of course exceptions to this rule, but generally speaking the doctor considers charitable gifts or donations

---

[1] Humble, J. G. (1966). *Brit. med. J.*, **1**, 156

towards medical or paramedical ventures the concern of the public.

My mind turns to another example, that of the Society of the Samaritans which was founded within recent years at the suggestion of an Anglican priest in London. He was aware of the many suicides and was convinced that if some help could be given to people when they were desperate to prevent them from taking their lives, many tragedies could be avoided. Volunteers were obtained, a telephone was provided and its number advertised and posted in every telephone booth so that any depressed person in need of help could ring any time of the day or night. Within a few minutes a Samaritan would be with him trying to see him through those critical hours and so put him in touch with a psychiatrist or other specialised person, depending on the circumstances which had led him to wish to take his life, in order to help him through his difficulties. It is claimed that this service has played a big part in reducing the number of these deaths. Be that as it may, it was conceived by a layman and is run free by lay volunteers although in reality it is a type of medical service.

Doctors show the same attitude, tantamount to one of superiority, towards medical auxiliaries, which they consider on a different or even lower plane than theirs. Fox, a former Editor of the *Lancet,* speaks of " the greater medical world " and shows how each division of the whole has a vital role to play in the actual recovery of the patient. We cannot do without the radiographer, the technologist, the nurse and the Red Cross voluntary worker. Whilst it would be out of place to weigh up the respective parts played by the many specialists in the wide field of medicine, we must never forget to recognise and respect the contribution of each one to the whole.

Freedom of Choice of Doctor

Should patients be able to choose their doctors? If we agree that the aim of medicine is to relieve or cure and that this can be attained through a doctor, this does not necessarily mean one of the patient's own choice. Because a doctor is employed in a service it does not signify that he cannot fulfil the purpose of medicine. But it is natural for man to choose someone who he thinks will best attain this object. He looks for a person whom he can trust, for he considers he is the one who will best help him. It does not follow that his choice is a wise one since individuals vary greatly in their reasons for selecting their doctors. When people seek a medical practitioner they look for one whom they think has not only the necessary skill and experience but also the personality that makes them feel confident. His reputation too helps in the final selection. Coming from the same part of the world, speaking the same language and belonging to the same social class all add in some indefinable way to this preference, rather like summing up a favourite horse in the paddock before a race. Its behaviour, personality and even the look in its eyes are taken into account. A man prefers to make his own choice and not to be regimented into accepting a doctor selected for him. It is not that he cannot be disciplined as in the army and other services, where the doctor is simply engaged on contract and these men and their families are told that he is the one who should attend to them. The principle of freedom of choice of doctor, admirable as it seems, is not an absolute necessity since relief or cure of an ailment can be achieved by these service doctors. Often the patient/doctor relationship that follows is a good and happy one. Much depends of course on the ability, understanding and other qualities of the doctor, the facilities at his disposal and on the opportunities his place of employment offers for consultation with specialists and consultants. But this does not mean that the patient, or the doctor himself, would not prefer freedom of choice. The patient looks upon the arrangement as an unnatural one. The service authority often has a much better idea of who is a good doctor than he has and who is likely to be " popular ", but its selection would not work in a society where the individual is free to choose.

The many factors that go into the choice of a doctor are difficult to list, but they may be compared with those that make a man choose his wife. He cannot say what prompted him to select a particular doctor. All that may be said is " I like this person. I felt I would be happy with him and no other."

Man is a complicated being with a behaviour indefinably deep, yet with a tendency to be sensible and logical. When selecting a doctor he may prefer one who is not likely to move in his own circle. Medical matters are personal and private and an individual may be embarrassed to meet his medical adviser regularly at the same social functions. Further certain disorders carry a stigma, such as, perhaps, venereal disease and a mental disorder.

In Africa we meet clans who still live in much the same way as they did for centuries and who have developed their way of life in accordance with the basic desires of man. In many ways they depict natural man at his best. The attitude of this society to its medical man is perhaps worth noting. All such African societies enjoy complete freedom in their choice of witchdoctor. Every person can choose whichever one he prefers and he can change to another " doctor " whenever he wishes. If he is not satisfied with the opinion or treatment he receives, he has no compunction in leaving one medicine man and consulting another. There is no obligation, as is customary amongst white patients, for the doctor who is being asked to take over a new client to seek permission first from his previous doctor. Natural man too pays for a cure. This is the standard practice amongst the Bantu and Negro races of Africa. This again seems reasonable. A person comes to a doctor to be cured and therefore he is prepared to pay for this. If he is no better he thinks the treatment was unsuccessful and therefore the medicine man is not entitled to a fee. From time to time we notice this feeling in a European patient who is slow to honour an account for an illness which did not respond to treatment. In contrast, when the treatment is effective in a very ill patient, it is surprising how quickly the money is paid. Although the African does not pay his medicine man a fee if he fails to cure, he accepts that he should pay for the herbs given as well as for any trouble the witchdoctor took on his behalf. He does not expect this medicine for nothing and is prepared to pay for it just as the European is accustomed to paying the chemist's bills. The patient appreciates that if a " doctor " travels a long distance to see him and if he is detained from his practice he should be adequately recompensed.

The European's attitude to service rendered by the doctor is reasonable as he accepts the principle that a charge should be made for each visit whether or not the medicine has achieved its object. He pays not for the cure but for the doctor's opinion and advice. He knows it may not always be right, realising that the correct diagnosis is not always possible. But he considers it just that he should pay for the doctor's advice as such in much the same way as he would pay for a lawyer's opinion. However, when his illness is chronic and the bills start mounting, the sick man begins to resist the ever increasing expenses. Again the layman agrees that the surgeon needs to be paid larger fees than other doctors and specialists. But he does not accept so readily a bill that runs into many pounds, especially when there are other costs to pay. This is known in most European countries and as a result some form of medical insurance or state medical service has resulted. It is not my purpose to discuss the merits and demerits of such services but merely to point out the patient's views on chronic and debilitating diseases or inconclusive surgical procedures which drain his reserves. He feels that all this is unfortunate and even perhaps unfair especially when he sees his finances diminishing on account of his ill health. Whilst he would prefer doctors of his own choice, the many expenses involved in modern procedure mean that he is more and more obliged to forgo this privilege. In most countries the state has been compelled to step in and help him out of his predicament. In a modern state freedom of choice of doctor or specialist is becoming less and less in

spite of great efforts by both the public and the profession to
retain this choice as far as possible.

A Doctor's Friends

The doctor makes many useful contacts in the society he
serves. Thus it can be expected that those who wield influence
because of their position or wealth might be ready or even wish
to help him as an expression of gratitude for his services. The
doctor may have saved the life of such a person and some
time later finds that through him he is able to get things done
that others are less successful in achieving. He finds that he
is popular, well-liked and has some good and trusted friends
in the community. Further his grateful patients go to almost
any length to help him. He even begins to believe that he must
be a really good person because so many people come to him.
He can get a child into a certain school, has his applications
accepted with little bother or permits granted when others
have difficulty in procuring them. This does not mean that the
doctor takes advantage of his position. The public is really
responsible. But in time the doctor learns that these are only
pseudo-friendships and if he takes the trouble to study his
relationship with these patients he soon realises it is purely
utilitarian, an expression of gratitude for what he has done.
Such friendships often lose their strength when he is unable
to cure some other member of the family. Relations are not
so warm or spontaneous. His invitations to tea and dinner
with the family diminish. All doctors experience this. It is
pleasant while it lasts, but the people concerned would never
have behaved in such a friendly way had a cure not been
established. The link between them is not a true association of
people wishing to be friends but one based on a service—often
a very good service and a desire to reciprocate in some way.

Just as the practising doctor has a ready means of introduction to a family circle and thus increases his circle of friends,
the opposite applies equally, for when he fails to please with

his remedies or his point of view, the patient may start to dislike him and his way of practice. He becomes a target for his wrath and this individual and his relations take every opportunity to besmear his name and reputation. This happens to every doctor when he has failed to achieve the desired results. He is blamed for not paying sufficient attention to his patient's complaints or not spending more time doing tests. He may have done everything possible and yet reached a wrong conclusion. Then, as is liable to happen, the patient may go to another doctor who happens to find the true nature of the illness. For instance, when the first doctor examined the patient, his urine may have been clear of glucose, yet on the next occasion the sample contained plenty. He is now told he has diabetes. He is grateful to the second doctor and blames the first. It may even happen that there was sugar in both specimens, but on the first occasion the nurse had forgotten to test it or had not done so properly. But unfortunately the first doctor has to take the blame. Had he found the sugar he would have gained a friend, but because he failed to detect it he lost one. I have known many individuals being annoyed or puzzled that a diagnosis was not made earlier and at every opportunity they let it be known that the doctor had let them down. On such occasions the doctor concerned must be extremely careful not to lose his temper or show his feelings. He must appear calm, dignified and even, if possible, show a sympathetic interest. If he argues or shows annoyance and upset at the patient's ignorance on such matters he may precipitate a bitter quarrel, even resulting in the patient consulting his lawyer and starting an action for damages against him. At this stage tempers must be avoided at all costs. Kindly words of explanation and an interest in the welfare of the patient often work miracles and avoid legal action. This then is the art of medicine, not only to please the patient in happy circumstances, but to calm him when he is bitter. Such a situation is likely to arise for any one of us sooner or later.

Who is to Blame?

I have watched the reactions of my patients, their close relatives and friends to their ailments and often wondered whether they were pleased with what I was doing for them. Did they understand the true situation when no one could help a person any longer? Could they see how seriously ill he was? There is nothing so good for a doctor as when all goes well with the patient, especially if he has been critically ill. The doctor has made the correct diagnosis early, instituted the specific remedy and recovery goes according to plan. Spirits are high! The doctor is on the crest of the wave. When he enters the hospital or the patient's home eyes beam at him; he is the hero; he feels elevated; he is competent, he had done good, perhaps even saved a life. As he walks up to the patient's bed his step is confident. The patient and his family are his friends. They will do anything for him. It is a pleasure to go into such a home at this stage in the illness. The patient is aware that the drugs have cured him, but had it not been for his clever doctor, how would he have known what to take? And so he usually gives the doctor credit. But there is a higher power than the doctor—God Himself, who directed him and so the doctor must not be too disappointed when the patient remarks casually that it is thanks to God that all has ended so well and happily. Still even then the doctor receives his share of appreciation.

And then there is the patient who is faring badly. The illness takes a downhill course. No matter what the doctor does for him he is not doing well. His condition may be deteriorating from a serious disorder which must end fatally. Yet the family resists the idea of an unhappy ending. They fear the worst but refuse to accept the situation. Each day that passes shows some deterioration. Disappointment is written all over the home. If only the doctor could work a miracle to stay the inevitable he would be happy! He must still visit the patient and show his interest and understanding of the situation. He is no longer treating only the patient but also the family. Often he manages tolerably well as the family see reason. But every now and then, as if to find a scapegoat for their misery, they seem to link him with the hopeless state of the patient, as if to take their minds off the afflicted one and turn them on the doctor. " Why does he not try a new injection or oxygen? " " We hear that Mr. So and So had exactly the same trouble and Dr. So and So gave this treatment. Don't you think you should try this? " " Don't you think you should ask for another opinion? " " Doctor—don't stop at any expense, try everything." And yet all is not hopeless for the doctor, especially if he has told the family the truth and the disorder has been correctly diagnosed. But if he has not recognised the nature of the illness early or the diagnosis is still not clear despite all tests, the situation is more critical. His visits are no longer pleasant. He realises that this is life and it cannot always be good for him. The patient dies. Perhaps the family were aware that the end had to come but almost subconsciously they link the death with the doctor. It is not so much an act of God although many accept that it was His will, but the doctor who did not know what he was doing. He was too slow and did not appreciate how ill the patient was. A few of the relatives do not forgive him although they declare it was " the will of God and we all go the same way." Then they add, " If only the doctor had come sooner or taken an X-Ray the result might well have been different."

Even then there is no telling how the family will behave. Man's reactions to particular situations can never be predicted with certainty. A patient may die and the doctor feel that the surviving husband or wife was not pleased with his services and then Christmas comes round and he is taken by surprise by the generous present he receives. Every doctor has experienced this. A patient dies or his condition deteriorates and the doctor feels that he has achieved nothing, yet members of the family speak gratefully of him. Perhaps their regard for the doctor can be explained as a transference of the love for

6

the departed to the person who was last at the bedside and tried to help him.

Everything is Green on the Other Side of the Fence

There comes a time in every practice when a cure cannot be effected and the sufferer begins to look elsewhere for help. At this stage the patient, and sometimes even the doctor, ceases to reason sensibly. In spite of competent opinion that everything possible has been or is being done, the sick person learns that in a bigger city nearby or in some far off capital there lives a gifted specialist with the ability to cure the disease from which he is suffering. There is of course good reason for the desire to consult someone else when the condition has not been diagnosed confidently but in a well established diagnosis of angina pectoris, asthma and certain other diseases there is often little justification for such journeys. Nevertheless every doctor must sooner or later face a request for his patient to go elsewhere.

No matter in what large centre the patient lives there is always some other city in which this remarkable opinion can be found. Even in London patients go to a city in Switzerland or Scandinavia. If it happens to be in a foreign country so much the better they feel. This does not mean that these cities do not have great medical men. But it is not scientific help that is being sought by these people. In reality they are looking for the mystical. When all has been done in the medical world or even before these means have been tried man resorts to the magical or spiritual cults practising medicine. He will always wish to try these means and it is useless attempting to stop him. Moreover it is quite remarkable to discover how often those whom we least expect to reason in this way support unorthodox opinion. Many people attending doctors revert to spiritual healers when faced with a critical illness. Often the higher a person is in the land and the further back he can trace his lineage the more liable he is to seek a " quack. ' I have tried to discover a reason for this and I wonder if it is because he links his social status with Divine power. Not long ago it was alleged that in one of the royal palaces in Europe unauthorised practitioners were called in to help a child for whom there was no hope of cure. The people of this country expressed their disappointment that such a dignified family should adopt such an unorthodox help. But this is just what should be expected. I once treated a noble lord whose ancestry could be traced back through many centuries and in the midst of his treatment he suddenly decided to consult the " box " an unscientific piece of apparatus in London about 5000 miles distant. In charge of the box is a quack who interprets its verdict. In the patient's mind was a firm belief linked with his spiritual past that he was not simply a physical being. The more regal or ancient a family, the firmer is its convictions that its ancestral association is real and can be consulted. From this it is but a step to try and contact this spiritual force in order to effect a cure.

Doctors and Politics

The doctor, like any other person, has his own likes and dislikes, his own attitudes to problems outside his field of work. Some are religious, perhaps an equal number indifferent and probably only a few are atheists. Some are very conservative and others again are " left " in their political views. At times they take part in politics with their fellow men. During a crisis they rally to support their country and are as patriotic as any other people. The doctor does his share in the growth and development of his country and is as vociferous as the rest. When it comes to hospital appointments, he may show the same likes, dislikes and prejudices that we meet in ordinary society. Thus until recently the medical profession has resisted the entry of women into medicine and until lately many London hospitals were extremely obstinate about accepting them. Prejudice is sometimes shown in medical appointments on the grounds of nationality, religion and background. Minority groups felt this prejudice when they came into contact with it and were disappointed with their colleagues. They considered they should be treated as doctors and that their religious beliefs should not matter. This preference of doctors for their own kind was revealed in relation to entrance to universities, posts in hospitals etc. These prejudices should not be confused with a doctor's qualities in his practice. He may well be a good doctor in spite of them. But it is disappointing to find members of such a great calling displaying such preferences. However, this is natural in man and we have to make allowances for a doctor's inconsistencies in life.

It is not easy for a doctor to practise in a community torn by political strife. Like other human beings he has his own views and may feel strongly about the political problems of his country. At times he may be known to belong to a political group which he serves actively. But he is generally careful not to mix his practice with politics and therefore is able to treat people in all walks of life holding all kinds of ideas. I think that in this his training has helped him to understand man's make up and to be tolerant. At times it can be very difficult to be tolerant, but, as a group, medical men show this quality as well as any other group, and some say, even better.

It is my impression that doctors are good employers. I have noticed that on the whole their nurses and secretaries generally work very well with them. There are the inevitable exceptions, but there usually seems to be a happy atmosphere in his practice or centre of research. This I believe is also due to his training which imbues him with tolerance towards other human beings.

For long I have pondered about the role doctors should take in political affairs and whether they would be more capable than the ordinary run of politicians who enter our parliaments today. At times I think they may well prove more able than legally-trained men because of their medical experience in human behaviour. Lord Malvern of Rhodesia has openly admitted his debt to medicine in his political career. He claimed that he tackled his political problems in the same way as he would when dealing with his patients. He assessed all the evidence and arrived at a conclusion just as he was accustomed to in reaching a medical diagnosis.

However, my advice to the practitioner who wishes to serve his community is to keep to medicine and avoid taking political sides. What counts in medicine is the patient and that the diagnosis made by the doctor should be the correct one, and in order to achieve this it is all important that there should be ease of communication between patient and doctor and that the patient should trust his medical practitioner. We have to be tolerant of the views of others. We realise that man's make-up, his physical being and his personality will always vary. There is always a certain percentage of idiots, geniuses, psychopaths, madmen, fascists and communists but mostly just ordinary people.

Medicine and the World Population Explosion

In his classic "An Essay on the Principles of Population " in 1798, the Rev. Thomas Malthus enunciated the rule that a population, if left, increased in a geometric ratio but the means of subsistence could only increase in an arithmetic one. The increase of population is limited by the means of subsistence. Further, the population increases when the means of subsistence increases. An excessive population follows a high birth and low death rate and man might consider reducing his fertility in accordance with the reduction in the mortality.

If medicine can claim to be responsible for saving lives through better recognition of disease, its better management and prevention, then we must consider whether the great increase in population in Asia and Africa is good; for unless economic opportunities exist for the newcomers the facilities for good and healthy living will become strained. With too many mouths to feed the standards drop and many people must grow up without an adequate education. Therefore it can be argued that medicine has not achieved its aim. The world is being made to suffer from this unprecedented increase in the number of people. But the aim of medicine is not basically concerned with the growth of the population of a country. Unless a woman approaches her medical adviser about having a child or more children when she may not be fit to bear them medicine itself is not concerned with the size of a family.

The birth rate of a country is far more a matter for ministers of religion, sociologists, economists or perhaps politicians. Individual members of the profession have become associated with birth control and family planning. It is true that there are many protagonists amongst doctors who actively assist this movement. Many of the devices used require the active participation of the doctor in their insertion. Thus in this instance members of the profession are actively concerned with the prevention of conception. Their participation does not interfere with the aim of medicine as life has not yet started nor is there actual sickness in the individual concerned. But when it comes to the performance of an abortion another set of circumstances arises and much bitter feeling results. Conception has taken place and life has begun. By performing an abortion the doctor is guilty of destroying a life, even though the foetus is not able to enjoy an independent existence until after 28 or more probably 30 weeks of life. If we accept that a foetus is a living being then an abortion is contrary to the principles of medicine. No one will deny that it is almost tantamount to killing a living child if life is terminated just before birth. A foetus of less than 12 to 16 weeks would not be viewed with the same concern as one close to term. Yet this is just a matter of degree. To me a week-old foetus is the same as one that is 35 weeks old and to destroy a product of conception even at so early a stage is an offence against mankind. Thus abortions that are not done on good medical grounds should not be permitted. The religious aspect, that of the Christian Church for instance, might well have influenced medical opinion in this respect.

We meet with the same aversion to interfering with a living product of conception among African tribes, amongst whom anyone, whether witchdoctor or otherwise, attempting to terminate a pregnancy is committing an offence and might even be accused of practising witchcraft. The natural and immediate reaction of most medical men is to disapprove of such an action. Doctors who do agree to it in their society, as in Sweden or Japan, have come to terms with their individual consciences. It can be argued that if a conception is ended as early as under 16 weeks, the foetus is not a living child and the procedure is comparable to no more than pulling out a plant from the soil and, as there are already too many people in the world, it is difficult to give each child born a proper chance in life. It may be said with good reason that because the profession is to a certain extent responsible for the increase in world population, it cannot shrug its shoulders over the consequences and take no part in the various attempts which aim at reducing the size of the family. Some hold the view that because of this the profession must also regulate the population increase, which is, in fact, a public health matter. Logical as this argument may appear I am not convinced that it is correct. Fundamentally the profession should be pleased with an increase in human life and look to the State to adopt proper measures to ensure that each person is able to enjoy a reasonable share of the resources available.

No Doctor is Poor in the Eyes of the Public

I remember some years ago being told that the average income of a doctor in England was only about £400 a year. But this included house-surgeons. How correct this figure was I cannot say. I was able to believe that many medical men were poor but I was not altogether convinced since I could not really say that I had yet met a poor doctor in actual practice. The public have come to look upon the medical profession as being better off than people of other professional groups. Many people even consider that they are some of the wealthier members of a community. I have tried at times to dispel this idea and pointed out that the doctor qualifies relatively late in life, then has to spend a few years in hospital at a low remuneration and thus has a much smaller span of active years in which to save and provide for his family than men in other callings who are generally able to start earning much earlier and have less to spend on their training, thus consolidating their positions much sooner.

None the less there seems little sympathy for the material status of the medical profession as a whole as people tend to look upon it as a better-off group. It is noticeable that where there is a more prosperous group amongst others envy follows and a certain amount of bitterness results. I have often heard it said that doctors are making " thousands " and in times of depression their wealth is believed to assume grandiose proportions. No matter how hard the doctor has worked for his earnings the disparity remains in the public eye. Although many reasons are advanced for the need of a reliable medical service this may have been an important factor in the desire of the politicians to control their earning powers.

Is it Right for a Doctor to make a Business of Medicine?

Is it right that a doctor should be allowed to earn more money than is reasonable for him and his family to possess? The question is complex. It is difficult to analyse the reaction of the general public to the earnings of a doctor, but my impression is that it is not opposed to some form of restriction, possibly because it still links disease with religion. True sickness was and still is regarded as a misfortune produced by influences that are difficult to understand, although the layman of today knows about bacilli, viruses and genetics. Is it not a fact that in every religion there is a belief in the spiritual powers of healing? Are not prayers offered in churches for the speedy recovery of the sick?

The association of religion and disease is very clear in the case of an African witchdoctor who is both a diviner and a herbalist. As a diviner he is a spiritual healer possessing the ability to contact the spiritual forces of the dead ancestors from whom he learns the cause of the sickness and what is required to propitiate the offended spirits, even though, in addition, he offers herbs and other medicines to cure the sickness. The Delphic oracle and the Asclepian cult in early Greece showed how man looked to a spiritual cause when struck by sickness, but from the time of Hippocrates the two disciplines, medicine and theology, became more and more separate and independent of each other.

Many members (probably the majority) of the medical profession are not opposed to earning as much as they want. They look upon their earnings as a reward or acknowledgment of their hard work and services. " Why," they argue, " should not the same apply to the doctor as to the lawyer, accountant, financier and writer : they are not restricted so why should we be?" "Are our wives and children not entitled to the benefits that money can give? Our children should be educated like the others and our homes should have the comforts and our wives the clothes that others have." The doctor, whether a surgeon, physician, general practitioner or specialist, who has a flourishing and even lucrative practice, likes to think that his recompense is a worthy recognition of his skill or high standard of practice and an appreciation of what he has done for the community.

In contrast to public reaction, an individual patient, as well as meeting his doctor's bill, not uncommonly gives him a handsome present to show his gratitude for what the doctor has done for him or his family. But in this way the patient is merely trying to express his personal gratitude in much the same way as he would give a present to anyone whom he wishes to acknowledge. He is not behaving inconsistently. He offers his personal thanks and token of appreciation for a special service rendered to him, although in principle he does not approve of doctors earning more money than is consistent with ordinary comfortable living.

One good result of envy amongst practitioners is that when a new specialist arrives in their midst some of them will support the newcomer at the expense of those in his speciality already established there. This gives him an opportunity to make a start and, as a result, there is a levelling of the other rival specialists. It is as if a man wants to restore the equilibrium reducing the wealth and superior status of those who have already made good in order to help a young doctor to find his feet. This little envy for one whose success they feel is greater than theirs keeps alive the spirit of competition and puts each man on his mettle as well as affording an immediate living to the newcomer.

Because of this rivalry between colleagues a doctor may feel the need of support for a certain project. For instance, he may require special apparatus, a research grant or financial aid in publishing his manuscript. Where is he to obtain the necessary means? Normally he should go to his own colleagues but he finds that amongst them he is likely to meet a rival or someone working in the same competitive field so his chances of obtaining their support are greatly lessened. Where it is possible he finds it preferable to ask a colleague far removed from the scene—one living in a different world to himself and thus not a competitor or else he seeks help from the lay public. Often such an approach wins him the necessary support. Thus when a doctor has to seek aid he stands a better chance of obtaining it from an outside person who is often much more willing to give him his full co-operation than his colleagues.

Human Frailties

What is the attitude of the medical profession to suicide? I have been told that every person has the right to decide whether he wishes to live or not. If one of the aims of medicine is to preserve life what should be the medical attitude to this? Some people are so unhappy for one reason or another that they feel there is no purpose in prolonging their misery. A man may have a cancer of the throat and life becomes unbearable. Who is to say that he should refrain from doing anything to shorten his life? Religion teaches that life is given to a person by God without his asking for it and therefore it is not his to take. The doctor is not concerned with this angle except, perhaps, in his personal capacity, if he is a religious man. Medically speaking, he does not attach a stigma to this act. In fact some doctors feel it is the individual's own affair. When we reflect on the causes for suicide we realise it is attempted when the mind is under stress or pressure and consequently it can be argued that the reasoning of the individual is not normal. Therefore when a doctor sees a patient with a suicidal tendency it is his concern to do whatever he can to prevent him from ending his life and to help him to adjust himself to his difficulties. He must preserve life and try to restore health. He must treat him in the same way as he would any other patient and do all he can to restore his mind to normal as well as attempting to remove or relieve any bodily disability from which he may be suffering.

If the medical profession is concerned with preventing a person from committing suicide how should its members behave towards certain risks or habits of their patients which may ruin or affect their well-being? Further, if it is known that a certain habit may damage health should a doctor adopt it himself knowing that the outside world looks to his profession for guidance on this matter? A minister of religion should set a good example to others. The tenets of religion are opposed to stealing or adultery and if ministers of religion preached against such acts but stole or lived with other men's wives, the public would tend to reject their faith even though its teachings should be accepted no matter what are the actions of the officials administering it. Then there is another aspect to this matter. When a man steals he deprives someone else and so the public conscience reacts against his act. But when a man smokes or eats to excess he harms himself and he is the one whose health suffers. Thus the same sanctions do not apply to the doctor as to the minister even though the former behaves as he wishes, ignoring the medical consequence of his acts. Scientists have shown that a clear association exists between smoking and lung cancer. There is a strong feeling that from the public health point of view action should be taken to eliminate the smoking habit. Prevention is always better than cure. Yet in spite of what seems to be the accepted proof, doctors continue to smoke. I have asked some of my colleagues the reason for this. The answers are revealing. Some fully appreciated the risk but felt that as they had to die of some disease eventually it might as well be lung cancer. Others again were not convinced of the truth, whilst yet others seemed little interested. Possibly most of them considered that as the habit concerned only the one who indulged in it and did not harm others as stealing did, it was purely a personal matter.

Other doctors answered me by saying that if they were to stop smoking why did people not give up driving motor cars which kill and injure so many? They carry a risk to both the driver and others. Therefore to stop this senseless loss of life he should not drive cars and at the same time should persuade others to give them up too. Yet we know this is false reasoning, for we simply must drive cars, which, apart from the pleasure afforded, provide an easy and rapid method of transport. We cannot live without taking some risks and driving a motor vehicle is one of those accepted necessities in life.

We might view overeating, especially of rich foods, as unwise since there is strong evidence that this predisposes to atheromatous thickening of the arteries, which in turn causes thrombosis of an artery such as the coronary. Yet many doctors, like many lay people, insist on enjoying fatty foods. We cannot legislate against the eating of rich food. To many people eating what they fancy is part of their existence and they will always want to be free to do as they choose. The same applies to smoking or drinking alcohol. Smoking gives personal pleasure to many people and seems to afford mental relief to anxious ones. At least to many people the habit is a help. Men's temperaments differ widely and medical reasons for giving up certain items of food, drink or other pleasures are never enough for some of them to accept. Whilst continuation of a particular practice may be followed by unpleasant results, yet they are not prepared to give up the material or mental advantages this custom affords them. Adultery, theft, murder and assault are bad in themselves and directly harm the innocent. Such actions are strongly condemned as antisocial by all. Thus the dogma of the Church is accepted readily, whereas all practices impairing health are not necessarily condemned out of hand by doctors. Just as the medical profession cannot legislate against suicide so it cannot take public action against habits and practices that may adversely affect the health of individuals. All it can do is put its views to the public as best it can and leave the individual to accept, reject or reserve judgment on them. If a doctor is asked for his advice he should give it in accordance with the principles of medicine.

Death

The doctor is intimately concerned with the preservation of life and the prevention of death, which is usually accompanied by much regret and distress on the part of the relatives. When life goes, the body is merely a lump of flesh and bone and is of no further use. Yet the doctor cannot treat it as something to be disposed of with all haste. To those concerned with the patient's departure the corpse still retains their respect and affection. To the wife it is the body of her husband, to a daughter that of her mother and father. Although dead the person is still alive both in mind and heart and will be remembered forever. To a great many people its soul or spirit is still alive and very much part of those living.

Today there still exists among all sections of society an involved funerary cult which reveals love and respect for the spirits of those departed. Among traditional Africans burial is accompanied by an elaborate ritual which must be carried out precisely lest the spirit be annoyed by the lack of respect and reveal its anger by causing illness or even death amongst the living members of the family. Even amongst Western people burial of the dead is accompanied by a religious service with much prayer. No matter how poor a person may be when some close relative dies he goes to no end of expense to give him a " decent burial ".

Reverence for the dead goes back to prehistoric days. From excavations in Europe we learn that before burying the dead, primitive man removed the skull and lower jaw, evidently attaching a special spiritual value to them. The head must have been regarded as the centre of reason and as containing the soul substance of man. Therefore it was considered essential to preserve the skull of his dead. Although primitive man feared the dead he was devoted to his own, believing that their spirits assumed supernatural powers which enabled them to influence and protect the living and even to punish them. This preservation of the skull indicated that primitive man practised a cult of the dead and probably prayed to them for protection, favour, help and perhaps for success in hunting.

Respect for the dead was still shown by the Egyptians much later in Neolithic times, when attempts were made to preserve the whole body after death. Not only was the body mummified but food was left in the tomb to sustain the dead man. This involved the belief in the immortality of the soul so strong in man.

It behoves a doctor to give the same consideration to the dead of others that he would give his own. He must be under-standing and respect the feelings of others. When a person dies and he knows the cause of death he can readily sign the death certificate which has to be produced before permission can be obtained for burial; but when he is not certain of the cause he is likely to find himself in a difficult situation. Many doctors in private practice sign certificates giving a cause of death even though they are not quite certain what it is. Should they, for the sake of science, request an autopsy or is it preferable not to argue with the relatives who more likely than not are going to refuse permission for this? I have found that if the doctor (or doctors) is reasonably certain of the cause of death and little information is likely to be gained from such a procedure, it is better to sign the certificate as people generally resent or even resist an autopsy being carried out on their relatives. The religious faith also has to be remembered. Autopsy is not permitted in certain faiths. On the other hand, if the doctor has no or very little idea of the cause of death he must not sign the certificate as there is the possibility that the person may have died from unnatural causes. A man drops dead in the street. He has not seen a doctor for some weeks or even months and after it is all over a doctor is called. This doctor should not issue the certificate although it is likely that the man died from coronary thrombosis or some vascular accident. Equally he must exercise caution when the circumstances surrounding the death are uncertain or suspicious.

It has been stated that a doctor in general practice should always try to have an autopsy when he is uncertain of the cause of death even though he has no reason to suspect unnatural causes or foul play. He is advised to do this so that he can learn and thus help others who may suffer from a similar condition. Again, this is a difficult matter on which to advise, but, knowing the reaction of the public of all races, I doubt whether the man in the street would agree to this procedure merely for the benefit of his doctor or ultimately to help mankind. Man naturally turns against dissection of the dead. On the other hand, the intention is different in a teaching hospital where medical students have to be taught tissue changes in disease. Thus if a patient dies in a teaching hospital an autopsy will generally be wanted and, even though the family of the dead person is opposed to this form of examination, the reason for it is a valid one. An autopsy in a teaching hospital is as essential for medicine as animal experimentation is. When a patient is admitted into a teaching hospital it should be on the understanding that an autopsy can be carried out in the event of death.

As an illustration of resistance to any interference with a dead body on religious grounds, I might usefully mention the scandal of the " missing heart " which I read about recently in the newspapers. In a country like Israel, where there is a strong objection to autopsy, it must be extremely difficult for the medical profession to procure sufficient material for teaching medical students the principles of medicine. There is a constant struggle between the religious bodies who resent autopsy operations and the medical profession which maintains that they are essential at times so that other lives may be saved by a closer study of lesions found in the viscera. Recently in Israel the wife of a rabbi died in hospital and as her body was prepared for burial it was discovered that the heart was missing. Upset relatives hurried to the hospital and demanded its return. It was duly handed over in a plastic bag, the hospital authorities explaining that it had been removed for massage prior to death in an endeavour to save the patient and as this occurred late at night after a very heavy day, the surgeon concerned was so tired that he had forgotten to put it back before sewing up the opening. The burial was now able to proceed.

" THE MOMENT OF DEATH "

Here we must ask ourselves when is a person dead. The Oxford English Dictionary defines death as " the final cessation of the vital functions ". Thus when the heart beat cannot be heard, all respirations have ceased (a mirror placed before the mouth shows no clouding), the pupils are fixed and dilated, the stare glassy and the jaw dropped, a verdict of death can be pronounced. Death can be said to have taken place when signs of *activity* cease completely in the cardiovascular, respiratory and nervous systems. At this moment the animus, vital spirit, call it what one will, has gone. But at " that moment of death " whilst activity as described above has been lost the tissue cells may be chemically and enzymatically intact even though life had departed and for a variable interval afterwards before degenerative changes take place in the cells. It is at this stage still possible to remove particular organs or tissues selected for surgical treatment and maintain them alive in an artificial environment for grafting or transplantation.

Premature pronouncements of death have been made in the past. Professor Keith Simpson (1967) an expert on forensic medicine, reminds doctors to be very careful when examining the body for signs of death. He stresses how necessary it is for the doctor to listen with his stethoscope for some minutes before pronouncing death, but even silence as he states may be found in drug comas, or in hypothermia the heart contractions being so faint as not to be detected with the ear, although electrical detectors will reveal that there is life. Hence a still electro-encephalogram is insisted upon in at least one American hospital so as to rule out any doubt before death is pronounced.

We know that a patient's heart may become arrested yet by massage and forced respiration it is possible to restore the circulation and the patient to life. But what if after the heart continues to beat there is evidence of severe brain damage or if the individual fails to recover consciousness. What should one do? The decision should be left to the doctor concerned. He might decide if there is no hope of restoring consciousness that he would cease all means of resuscitation so allowing the patient to pass on. If the patient has suffered serious brain damage after being restored to consciousness, should the heart suddenly fail at a later date, he might decide not to resort again to resuscitation.

With the many strides made in surgery it is now possible to graft tissues from the freshly dead with those who are in great need of these parts and so the " moment of death " has a legal significance when suitable organs or tissues are to be removed from a donor at the time of his death. It is obviously important that the material be excised before degenerative changes have set in. If in an effort to procure the sample in its best condition the operator removes it before that " moment of death " he would be committing an assault and might be faced with an accusation of having precipitated death (Simpson, K. (1967) *Abbotempo* Book 3, page 22). A proposal was put forward for dis-

7

cussion at a recent international conference that it should not be unlawful for material to be removed for treatment purposes if it was taken after death or whilst the tissues were being maintained in a living state. On the one hand there is that bodily death which medical men have always known and on the other and distinct from it a " death " in which cells and their enzymes are still viable, life in them only being maintained by artificial help. My own reaction to this would be that even if the heart beat is maintained only by artificial means no organ should be removed for organ transplantation since a vital function is still in existence and there is life, however tenuous.

The Examination

On occasions I have heard members of the public grumbling that a doctor has charged them a big fee when all he did was to ask a few questions without even examining them. Many doctors will agree that at times a patient objects to a fee because the examination was so brief. Some people are pleased with a doctor if he spends an hour or more with them. I have heard patients speak well of a doctor because he gave them so much of his time. This is understandable and reasonable that a patient should feel that the longer the doctor spends on the examination the greater his interest in him and the less likely he is to overlook something serious. He is considered more careful. However, we should not form any hasty conclusion for the length of time is not necessarily the criterion of a good examination. Much depends on the nature of the complaint and the experience of the doctor. A skin specialist may recognise the nature of a lesion almost at a glance and a tropical diseases expert can spot a leper as he walks into the consulting room. There is no need for him to spend a long time with such a patient. On the other hand, one with dyspepsia requires far more questioning, a careful physical examination and possibly a barium meal investigation. A practitioner who has seen a certain ailment regularly would detect it more readily than one who meets it only infrequently.

We might ask what is meant by examination. Does it entail the taking of details about the patient's complaint, followed by a physical examination and then by testing his specimens and perhaps other laboratory tests? What is the definition of an examination? According to the Oxford English Dictionary it can have several meanings. Perhaps the nearest to what I am seeking is " the formal interrogation of a witness in an enquiry by inspection ". For instance, would one accept merely looking at the patient if he has an obvious florid skin eruption? Is it necessary to go through the formal procedure in every case? I believe both the doctor and the patient must be reasonable in this matter and the time taken over the examination must be long enough to satisfy both parties that the diagnosis is clear (or not clear as the case may be) and the patient under-stands what is wrong with him and what he has to do. Nowa-days especially, the public is more fully aware of the scientific advances in medicine and what tests may be expected. In all cases, except in those in which the condition is obvious, the doctor must conduct a proper examination. At all costs he should never tell a patient that he has a malignant growth, tuberculosis of the lungs, leukaemia or some other serious disorder before he has carried out the recognised and special procedures which the public expect of a clinician. After he has taken a careful history and conducted the physical exam-ination, if he considers it wise or appropriate in that particular case, he can mention to the patient what is on his mind and it is for that reason that he is instituting the necessary investiga-tions or referring him to a specialist.

CHARACTERISTICS OF THE PROFESSION

Conservatism

THE medical profession is the most conservative of all professions. It tends to resist change more than any other group
of people and then accepts it reluctantly. Before it agrees
it has to be convinced that it is for the better and in the interest
of the patient. This is understandable as we have learnt of
catastrophic treatments in which many people have lost their
lives, although the trials concerned may have been undertaken
in good faith and with the sincere belief that the treatments were
the right ones. For instance, we all know that a number of
people died of tuberculosis as a result of B.C.G. vaccine which
was first introduced in France in about 1906. We can appreciate the horror these fatalities produced in the minds of the
public. The profession has to exercise caution and dare not
follow blindly every new suggestion. It has to remember too
that there are dishonest men who, for gain or fame, are willing
to risk the patient's life on some ill-founded, unauthorised
medical procedure.

Yet we can err by being too conservative. It does not matter
which field is concerned, surgical, medical, obstetrical or public
health, the profession refuses to move an inch unless it can
be convinced that the procedure is safe. Personal feelings,
rivalries and jealousies, all the frailties of human nature, enter
into many of the reasons for resisting a new procedure or treatment. Perhaps the worst example of this conduct by the
medical profession was displayed in 1865 when Lister announced his new technique of antiseptic surgery. In spite of the
important experiments with all the scientific requirements for
exactitude carried out by Pasteur and Lister's own well-

documented observations, the British doctors bitterly opposed the new concept. No doubt envy influenced many of those opposed to Lister's deductions that germs caused hospital sepsis and that gangrene could be eliminated by the application of carbolic acid to the normal wound. The leading surgeons, notably those in London, steadfastly refused to be convinced, despite the fact that French and German surgeons had already adopted Lister's methods. When he came to London from Edinburgh, at least six years after announcing his revolutionary observation in the *Lancet,* he met with a cold, unfriendly, unco-operative reception from the medical fraternity.

All through our medical history the profession has resisted change. Doctors seem to grow accustomed to a train of medical thought even when there is much evidence to show that it is incorrect ; they gladly continue in the old way. What better example can be given than that of Galen's hypothesis? His concept of the circulation through a most extraordinary route lacked anatomical proof. According to this postulation the vital spirit, which was inhaled, passed from the right to the left ventricle through invisible pores. For more than 1,400 years this was accepted by the profession and the Church and anyone who doubted it was proclaimed a heretic. Michael Servetus, a Spanish theologian and physician, was burnt at the stake in Geneva in October 1553 because he doubted the Galenic concept and described the pulmonary circulation.

The profession never seems to learn its lesson, perhaps because man remains the same and it is his nature to conform and to oppose change. As new ideas continually intrude into the daily routine of the medical practitioner it is hoped that the profession will become more reasonable about their acceptance.

The Fear of Losing Patients

Rarely can a doctor bear to see his patients leaving him and going elsewhere for aid. It implies a loss of confidence in his ability to treat them and although not in itself a realistic threat to his practice perhaps he feels he is in danger of losing it, which of course is of great concern to him. So no matter how difficult it is to keep certain patients he makes every effort to please them. He does his best not to upset the good relationship between him and his clientele. It is extraordinary to what lengths a doctor will go to ensure that his patients will not leave him.

In my many years of intimate contact with the general practitioner I have found few who were pleased to call in a second opinion. It is quite true the patient and his family often have little idea of the true position or are able to judge when another opinion should be sought. An illness may be acute and threaten life or it may be long, painful and costly and then naturally those concerned have recourse to outside help. It is not a reflection on the part played by their family doctor or on his skill. In spite of his knowledge and the regard they have for him they just want to be sure that nothing more can be done. Sometimes, it is true, a patient may have lost confidence in his medical attendant. For various reasons he begins to doubt his competency and may demand another opinion. Again the sick person may have heard that another doctor is skilled in treating his particular complaint. He may have built up a reputation for that very disease from which he is suffering and he feels he must see him even though his general practitioner is surprised at this wish.

Many a practitioner is loth to call in a second opinion unless circumstances force him to do so. He generally feels his ability is being questioned. At the back of his mind lurks the fear that if a diagnosis or treatment other than his is suggested the patient will leave him and his livelihood will be threatened: so if he has to ask for another opinion he refers the patient to a consultant in another part of the country miles away so his " mistake " will be minimised and he remains in charge of the case. He fears a distant consultant less than a local one.

If the doctor thinks realistically he will call in a second opinion, perhaps not with alacrity, but because it is expected of him. Even the public knows this weakness. I have often been approached by a patient wishing to see me. When I explain that I must have a letter from his doctor he always replies, " but I do not wish to hurt my doctor." He would rather go behind the practitioner's back than offend him; he cannot summon the courage to ask for a letter of introduction.

The position is much more simple amongst the traditional African people where no consultation occurs between witch-doctors. We in the Western world are a stage further. In spite of the natural feelings of man we do not permit secrecy in the use of remedies and when the doctor or his patient decides that progress is not being achieved fast enough the former should seek a fresh point of view from one of his colleagues. The principle of consultation has been accepted by medical men from the time of Hippocrates. A wise doctor knows when to suggest a consultation. He should try to anticipate the patient's desire for such. He must judge the propitious moment when to suggest it. He should do this as soon as he sees some doubt, uncertainty or concern on the part of the patient. In this we see the artist at his best. It is no longer the scientist who counts but the man who knows human nature. It is not an easy situation and it calls for understanding and sympathy on the part of the doctor. But the practitioner who can judge when to seek a second opinion, even if in his opinion there is no need for one medically, will not lose that patient but win his confidence.

For 'tis a Green-eyed Monster

Whatever course we choose in our medical work, whether as a doctor devoted to the science of medicine or one who practises amongst the public it is by no means easy. Nothing comes without effort. All is not smooth for sooner or later the enthusiast is bound to meet with human difficulties. No matter how he tries to avoid it opposition arises. He never knows who will become his opponent or who will object to his achievements in his particular field. He feels that if only this person were not in the picture all would be perfect, but if his rival disappears another takes his place. I have known the doctor so frustrated by this rivalry that he gives up his practice and goes elsewhere. I well remember my professor of surgery telling me that as soon as a doctor becomes very successful envy is aroused and difficulties follow. It does not matter in which aspect he excels, some colleague will be displeased and try to thwart him. I do not know of a single instance in which a successful individual has escaped.

This envious reaction provoked by another's success is not confined to the clinician or doctor in actual practice but is equally bitter among the academics of a university. It matters not whether a doctor works for his living in private practice, is employed in a full-time hospital appointment or engaged in medical research, any success, great or little, always evokes envy on the part of someone. It may be someone fairly far removed from his place of work, in another town miles away perhaps or it may be one of his so-called best friends. But he becomes aware of it. The doctor should not be too disappointed. Jealousy is part of man's nature just as love is. It is merely a means by which he protects himself. It cannot be divorced from his make-up. It is no use protesting that it is not in keeping with professional people who belong to such a fine calling as medicine. Man is still man whatever his work in life. Jealousy exists in many other sections of society even among religious groups. However if the one who suffers it is realistic and tries to be understanding he can make allowances for it. Mostly such jealousies can be discarded and their victims emerge unscathed. They very seldom amount to more than feelings of envy and the person who feels them takes no active steps to harm the other doctor. He may belittle his success, question his knowledge, imply that his work is not up to standard and seize every opportunity to criticise his diagnoses. In reality these are mere pin-pricks, annoying as they are, to the person who evokes this jealousy. It is best for him to ignore these reactions and push ahead on his set course. No good will come out of bitter arguments and it is difficult to corroborate the information that comes to him through second and third parties. Further by letting it upset him or by brooding over it he may allow his output and standard of work to suffer. He has at all costs to maintain that happy and confident frame of mind so conducive to good productive thought. I must admit that occasionally an innocent man becomes the victim of a jealous rival. He may find himself transferred to another station or lose a contract in his practice. Once a jealous doctor takes action there is no limit to what he will do, but as I have pointed out, such instances are rare. Ordinary feelings of jealousy, which find expression, can be safely disregarded.

I have mentioned all this for the benefit of the young doctor starting off on his career. I cannot see the reason for only extolling the great and glorious features of the medical profession. Every doctor should know its defects and weaknesses as well as its strength and virtues. He should also be aware of the basic nature of man and know that the doctor is no different from other men in this regard. He will know what to expect not only in others but in himself as well. He could develop the art of being able to recognise this feeling of envy in himself, learn to control it and to pursue only positive, useful and creative ideals.

Doctors are not more jealous than other men, but it is often said that the degree of envy amongst them is greater than in any other profession. I once discussed this matter with a judge who was particularly interested in our profession as his son is a doctor. He stated that such envy did not exist to the same extent amongst members of the bar. He remarked that advocates could argue against each other in court, but once outside, all was forgotten and they were as friendly as ever. It is possible that a doctor would be more likely to give free vent to his feelings than a lawyer whose training has taught him caution in expression. I cannot believe that the success of a barrister will not evoke feelings of envy in one of his colleagues.

A doctor's patients discuss their illnesses and treatment with their friends and when a cure has not been effected there is always the risk that they will change their practitioner in favour of one praised by these friends. A failure to cure may so easily lead to loss of reputation and consequently of some of his practice and thus a diminution of his income. He always has the fear that he may be held responsible for a failure and always lurking in the background is the even greater one that he might be sued for negligence. The doctor may not think of this consciously in his daily practice but subconsciously the fear is there. He comes to place undue stress on his successes or failures. Yet I know of no sociological study which proves that the medical profession is basically different in its attitude towards its colleagues than any other profession. I am reminded of the saying, " No man likes his fellow artist."

Doctors like Praise

Most people enjoy words of praise: they soothe the heart, warm the marrow and so it is difficult in this matter to compare one professional group with another. But perhaps I am correct in saying that the doctor loves to hear kind things said of him more than any other professional group. To him it is a form of acknowledgment of his work, a return for help he has given and, as he depends on the attitude of other human beings towards him, he is very receptive to a little praise, cautious as he is not to boast about his skill or successes. He is a modest person in this. He knows better than most the frailty of life and human nature and the uncertainty of the next day. He knows he cannot always cure and accepts this as inevitable. He realises that many of his patients will be displeased when recovery does not go off well, errors may be made and he might well be blamed for not recognising the answer to a particular problem. So, as if to compensate for this uncertainty, he is grateful for the few words of praise which comfort him and restore his confidence. They reassure him that his reputation is good and that people think kindly of him and make up for the disappointments he has to face.

8

THE MEDICAL CODE

The Hippocratic Oath and the Declarations of Geneva and Helsinki

THE ANCIENT Hippocratic Oath remains the basic ethical code upon which medical practice is founded today and its principles and concepts are incorporated in the framework of constitutions of world medical councils. Many graduates of medicine take the Oath (or the more recent Declaration of Geneva which was founded upon it) although not everyone is obliged to swear to it on qualification. So as to allow one to study the Hippocratic Oath and the Declaration of Geneva both are quoted in full.

The Oath of Hippocrates

" I swear, by Apollo Physician, by Asclepius, by Health, by Panacea and by all the gods and godesses, making them my witnesses, that I will carry out, according to my ability and judgment, this oath and this indenture. To hold my teacher in this art equal to my own patients; to make him partner in my livelihood; when he is in need of money to share mine with him; to consider his family as my own brothers, and to teach them this art, if they want to learn it, without fee or indenture; to impart precept, oral instruction, and all other instruction to my own sons, the sons of my teacher, and to indentured pupils who have taken the physician's oath, but to nobody else. I will use treatment to help the sick according to my ability and judgment, but never with a view to injury and wrong-doing. Neither will I administer a poison to anybody when asked to do so, nor will I suggest such a course. Similarly

I will not give to a woman a pessary to cause abortion. But I will keep pure and holy both my life and my art. I will not use the knife, not even, verily, on sufferers from stone, but I will give place to such as are craftsmen therein. Into whatsoever houses I enter, I will enter to help the sick, and I will abstain from all intentional wrongdoing and harm, especially from abusing the bodies of man or woman, bond or free. And whatsoever I shall see or hear in the course of my profession, as well as outside my profession in my intercourse with men, if it be what should not be published abroad, I will never divulge, holding such things to be holy secrets. Now if I carry out this oath, and break it not, may I gain for ever reputation among all men for my life and for my art, but if I transgress it and forswear myself, may the opposite befall me."[1]

The Oath is remarkable for its depth of understanding; it defines what is expected of a doctor so that he may maintain a happy relationship with his patient and at the same time it lays down certain principles of medicine.

There is a preamble in the Oath dealing with the financial support of the teacher of medicine by his qualified pupil under certain circumstances; the new graduate promises to teach children of his instructor as though they were his brothers and to share his livelihood with him in the event of necessity. It would seem that the teacher of medicine would be helped if necessary by those doctors he trained. Perhaps the student of those days could not afford to pay much for his training but once he was qualified and was in a secure position he promised to assist the one who had helped him. This no longer applies today as the system of training is different. There is an understanding amongst some of those training to be witchdoctors that the first ox received in fees to be paid to the teacher since there is often no fee for his instruction.

The Original Oath began with the words, " I swear by Apollo Physician, by Asclepius, by Health, by Panacea and

[1] Jones, W. H. S. (1948). *Hippocrates.* English Translation, p. 299. Heinemann, London.

by all the gods and godesses, making them my witness." This has been interpreted by some as showing that Hippocrates belonged to the Asclepian cult and therefore he accepted the magico-religious practices and causes of disease. This may have been the case, but others argue that the Oath itself does not contain a single word to support this allegation. In any event this ancient cult may have been the doctor's religion just as Christianity may be his faith today.

Another passage has proved a stumbling block and has been criticised by many of the medical profession: " I will not use the knife, not even, verily, on sufferers from stone, but I will give place to such as are craftsmen therein." This might be interpreted as meaning that the Hippocratic school was opposed to surgery, but at this point, we might remember that surgery may have been regarded not as medical but as belonging to other " craftsmen." It was at that time a part of treatment outside the scope of the physician.

The main substance of the Oath is of great interest and I should like to stress the following points :

" I will use treatment to help the sick according to my ability and judgment."

" Into whatsoever houses I enter I will help the sick."

The Oath thus infers that the doctor is to help a sick person and it is in this context alone that we might accept the aims or purpose of medicine, a view to which I have always subscribed. The next passage supports my contention that it is the duty of the doctor to preserve life:

" Neither will I administer a poison to anybody when asked to do so, nor will I suggest such a course. Similarly I will not give to a woman a pessary to cause abortion, but I will keep pure and holy my life and my art." The Oath is clear about the attitude of the profession to secrecy:—

" And whatsoever I shall see or hear in the course of my profession, as well as outside my profession in my intercourse with men if it be what should not be published abroad, I will never divulge, holding such things to be holy secrets."

The meaning of the words in the Oath " from abusing the bodies of man or woman, bond or free " is given in other versions of the Oath as seduction or illicit sexual intercourse (see *Percival's Medical Ethics* edited by Chauncey, D. Leake (1927), Baltimore. Williams & Wilkins Company, p. 213: also British Medical Association, *Members Handbook* (1965), p. 54.)

It is worth remarking that the Oath makes no reference to fees or doctor's charges. It speaks of the doctor keeping " pure and holy both my life and my art." Again in a later passage it says " and I will abstain from all intentional wrongdoing and harm, especially from abusing the bodies of man and woman, bond or free." There is no reference in these words to fees charged for his service. This omission is significant as the Oath is not concerned with how he is employed or from whom he receives his pay. What matters is that he should keep pure and holy and not transgress in this aspect of medical practice.

The Declaration of Geneva must be quoted in full. It is in the main much the same as the Hippocratic Oath. As a result of the perpetration of crimes against the human being and lapse from the Hippocratic Oath by members of the profession during the Second World War, it was felt necessary for a more modern revaluation of the old Oath. Therefore in 1947 the World Medical Association produced the Declaration of Geneva which aims at uniting the medical profession into a single brotherhood. It stresses that the patient is the first consideration and recognises that secrets confided to the doctor must be respected. It reminds him of the utmost regard he must show for human life from the time of conception. In other words he is obliged to preserve life. The Declaration calls upon the doctor to do all in his power to maintain the honour of the medical profession and when called to a patient not to permit considerations of religion, nationality, race, politics or social standing to interfere with his duty and to base upon it an international code of medical ethics for adoption both in peace or in time of war.

THE GENEVA DECLARATION

(Extracted from the B.M.A. Handbook (1965) p. 55)

" At the time of being admitted as a member of the medical profession I solemnly pledge myself to consecrate my life to the service of humanity:

" I will give to my teachers the respect and gratitude which is their due;

" I will practise my profession with conscience and dignity;

" The health of my patient will be my first consideration;

" I will respect the secrets which are confided in me;

" I will maintain by all the means in my power the honour and the noble traditions of the medical profession;

" My colleagues will be my brothers;

" I will not permit considerations of religion, nationality, race, party politics or social standing to intervene between my duty and my patient;

" I will maintain the utmost respect for human life from the time of conception, even under threat; I will not use my medical knowledge contrary to the laws of humanity;

" I make these promises solemnly, freely and upon my honour."

The English text of the International Code of Medical Ethics is as follows:—

Duties of Doctors in General

"A doctor must always maintain the highest standards of professional conduct.

" A doctor must practise his profession uninfluenced by motives of profit.

The following practices are deemed unethical:

(a) " Any self-advertisement except such as is expressly authorised by the national code of medical ethics.

(b) " Collaborate in any form of medical service in which the doctor does not have professional independence.

(c) " Receiving any money in connection with services rendered to a patient other than a proper professional fee, even with the knowledge of the patient.

" Any act, or advice which could weaken physical or mental resistance of a human being may be used only in his interest.

" A doctor is advised to use great caution in divulging discoveries or new techniques of treatment.

" A doctor should certify or testify only to that which he has personally verified."

Duties of Doctors to the Sick

" A doctor must always bear in mind the obligation of preserving human life.

" A doctor owes to his patient complete loyalty and all the resources of his science. Whenever an examination or treatment is beyond his capacity he should summon another doctor who has the necessary ability.

" A doctor shall preserve absolute secrecy on all he knows about his patient because of the confidence entrusted in him.

" A doctor must give emergency care as a humanitarian duty unless he is assured that others are willing and able to give such care."

Duties of Doctors to Each Other:

" A doctor ought to behave to his colleagues as he would have them behave to him.

" A doctor must not entice patients from his colleagues.

" A doctor must observe the principles of ' The Declaration of Geneva ' approved by the World Medical Association."

Doctor and Citizen

What should be our attitude to the moral issues that may arise from the action of men in the prosecution of warfare, chemical, biological or in a military force?

I should like to quote one who is concerned with this point. " Doctors have struggled for centuries to eradicate the very diseases now being considered for possible release on whole populations. Today doctors may be instrumental in the spread of epidemics as acts of war. How does this square with the Declaration of Geneva ' I will maintain the utmost respect for human life . . . even under threat ' or ' I will not use my medical knowledge contrary to the laws of humanity '? How does a doctor using his medical knowledge to produce a more infectious strain of anthrax reconcile his work with Hippocrates' precise injunction, ' First do no harm '? Where indeed does he draw the line?"[1] This is a difficult problem but one that would not arise if it were realised that Hippocrates in his Oath concerned himself with the conduct of a practising doctor towards his individual patient. Hippocrates was not concerned with humanity at large or with nations or peoples as such, only with the doctor and his responsibility to the sick individual seeking his help. This is strictly a discipline existing between a doctor and a sick person and once this relationship has been established he is in honour bound to aid and not harm him. But whatever the doctor did outside this specific doctor-patient relationship does not appear to have concerned Hippocrates. There is no reason therefore why a doctor should not fight and die for his country or lend his medical knowledge for its defence. In fact it has been his lot to ensure the fitness of the army for the final battle and by so doing he is an active participant in the armed forces. In the same context the medical scientist may improve the bacteriological weapons upon which his country depends for its continued safety.

Not to Divulge

Doctors are silent about their patients' complaints and there is little careless talk about confidential matters. Not only do they not reveal details of their patients' troubles to lay people but are equally cautious when talking to their colleagues. It is only natural for a medical man to talk about diseases to other

---

[1] Macdonald, J. B. (1967). *Lancet,* **1,** 563.

doctors when he sees them. They talk " shop " as is only to be expected and disclose that they are seeing a good deal of diarrhoea, liver disease or indeed anything that interests them, but they are always careful not to mention names or speak about anything that is better not told to anyone. Therefore they are most selective in what they say, where they say it and to whom. They do not spread medical gossip. By the time they have qualified they have learnt to respect matters of a personal nature. A doctor is like a minister of religion in this and I can only rarely recall one speaking out of turn.

Every doctor always carries with him the thought that he has been told something confidential. He hardly sees a case without hearing something which is told in confidence. Indeed when a patient relates the history of his complaint he does so with the tacit understanding that this is only for the doctor's ears. This does not mean that he would necessarily object if his doctor revealed the nature of his complaint. For instance when he belongs to a medical aid society the doctor is required to divulge the diagnosis before it meets his expenses. The patient knows this and is prepared for it to happen. So it would not be true to say that the doctor is always given the case details in absolute secrecy. Yet very few doctors betray the confidences of their patients, especially about any matter that has a personal or social stigma associated with it. He is most unlikely to mention details about venereal disease or mental disturbances in a patient to other people when these matters are not absolutely secret.

There are occasions when a doctor is never prepared to reveal information. If for example, a woman has had an illegal abortion and he knows who did it he would look upon this information as given to him in absolute trust and would not reveal who committed the offence when asked to do so. The Hippocratic Oath makes this attitude to secrecy very clear:—" And whatsoever I shall see or hear in the course of my profession as well as outside my profession in my intercourse with men, if it be what should not be published abroad, I will never divulge, holding such things to be holy secrets."

At the Third General Assembly of the World Medical Association held in London in October, 1949, an International Code of Medical Ethics was established and it had this to say about secrecy:—" A doctor shall preserve absolute secrecy on all he knows about his patient because of the confidence entrusted in him."[1] The doctor looks upon himself as his patients' confidant and will not want to disclose the matter to anyone, not even to a relative unless it is in the patient's interest that he does so and provided he knows that what he is revealing cannot harm the patient or place him in an embarrassing situation. Indeed he could be sued for divulging verbally or in writing any matter concerning his patient's illness without his prior consent or, in the case of a minor, that of his guardian. However, a doctor can be summoned to court, where, under oath, he is obliged to reveal matters ordinarily considered a breach of professional secrecy. Thus in the court of law he is like any other person and must go when summoned. Failure to do so would amount to contempt of court and he could be imprisoned. Any party may call on any person who has the knowledge to testify before it. Thus whilst any party to a suit may call on a doctor as a witness, only the court itself can require him to testify. Even then the doctor may prefer not to betray his patient's confidence even if he knows he will be sent to prison for this.

The wish for secrecy about an individual's illness is recognised too by the witchdoctors in Africa. Amongst them we find the same ethical code as in other societies. Man objects to discussions about personal matters. Medical consultations take place in an atmosphere of confidence and the sick person naturally expects his sensibilities to be respected. It is therefore hardly necessary for any promise or oath to be taken on such

[1] Masters, N. C. & Shapiro, H. A. (1966). *Medical Secrecy and the Doctor-Patient Relationship*. Balkema, Capetown.

a matter since it is part of man's make-up to respect this desire for secrecy. However, it can be very serious if a matter is revealed even unintentionally. A stray word, an indiscreet phrase or even a gesture may reveal a love affair and perhaps break up a marriage or a close friendship or invite the arm of the law. Therefore a doctor's safest course is to maintain silence unless under oath in court.

It may be argued that when a patient calls in a doctor and relates his story the doctor is violating his confidence if he reveals it to someone in a laboratory or X-Ray department. Here he is not being unethical since he is merely continuing or extending the consultation with those who can help to diagnose the complaint and this course of action is accepted by the patient.

Even death does not alter the confidence placed in an individual's medical attendant. The patient may have suffered from a disease which may adversely affect the standing of his family and it is assumed that he would not want to impair the family reputation. Whether he has or not, whether the information is of historical importance or not, his trust should not be broken. All that he learns about his patient and his family whilst attending them is confidential. But a doctor who is not personally concerned with this trust can use such information historically provided he obtains it in the conventional archival way.

Sometimes circumstances arise in which it is difficult to know what to do. I remember sitting in the dining room of one of the large hotels of a city, when two men came in, sat down and ordered a meal. I was certain one was a leper. The more I looked at him the more concerned I was that a man with his complaint should be at large in a public place. But I decided that as he had not consulted me I was not in a position to say anything to anyone. Had he done so I would have had to notify the public health authorities, since in the country in which I was practising this is a notifiable disease. Further there was always the possibility that my diagnosis was incorrect. Without carefully examining a person no one has the right to make a diagnosis. What would I have done if that man had been covered in a classical smallpox rash? There my attitude might have been different. Firstly the life of the person himself would have been in danger, so, if I went up and told him that he might have smallpox, he might have been grateful for having his attention drawn to the need for seeking medical aid immediately. On the other hand the leper would think I was interfering with his freedom and resent this.

On another occasion I was faced with a problem which involved a member of my own family. One of my unmarried relations was going out with a man whom I had seen a few years before with intermittent claudication. He apparently had occlusive vascular disease. Should she be warned that he had an incurable disease? I said nothing. The man was my patient and I had no right to divulge this information. Of course had it come to me outside my profession, I would have had every right to pass it on to the girl. In that event I would have had no bond with the sick person and it would have been my duty as an individual to draw her attention to his ill health in the same way as I would if he had had some other defect, such as an addiction to alcohol or had misbehaved in some way. It so happened that he did not marry her.

I also recall treating a man who had attempted to end his life. He was a homosexual. He was a fine scholar and had applied for a position in a teaching institute. Someone who knew of his tendencies had warned the headmaster who came to see me about this application. My conscience was troubled. Might he not interfere with one of the boys in the institution? What was I to do? I decided that I had no authority to reveal anything about my patient and he was given the appointment.

What should a doctor do if, during the examination of a patient who has consulted him, he discovers or is strongly suspicious that this person is a criminal or perhaps even a murderer? The police may be seeking him but are not aware of his identity. Should the doctor lift the telephone and inform them that he has found the culprit? This is a most difficult situation. Is the doctor to maintain his professional secrecy? Is he to consider himself outside the arm of the law and withhold this information? If he does not tell can he expect police protection in the future in the same way as any other member of the State? By maintaining silence he is laying himself open to legal prosecution.

In Halsbury's Laws of England (third edition, vol. 26, paragraph 10, page 11) the position is summed up as follows:—

" *Obligation to give evidence.* The relationship between a medical practitioner and his patient does not excuse the former, whatever medical etiquette may require from the obligation, if called upon, to give evidence in a court of law. He is in the same position as any other person who is not specially privileged in this respect by the law. He may be summoned to give evidence in civil or criminal cases, and is liable to be punished for contempt of court if he neglects to attend.

He may be asked to disclose on oath information which came to him through his professional relationship with a patient; and if the question is not inadmissible on other grounds, he may be committed for contempt of court if he refuses to answer."

According to the same authority, in a footnote to paragraph 10 the following is said:—

" (i) A medical practitioner, who in the course of treating a patient under a national scheme for dealing with venereal disease ascertained that the patient was suffering from venereal disease, could be compelled to give evidence to that effect, although the statutory regulations applying to the scheme enjoined absolute secrecy on the medical practitioner (*Garner* v. *Garner* (1920) 36 T.L.R. 196; cf. now the National Health Service (Venereal Diseases) Regulations, 1948, S.I. 1948 No. 2517). Hawkins, J., when summing up to the jury in *Kitson* v. *Playfair* (1896), *Times,* 28th March, said ' I can quite understand a case, especially in a civil case, where a doctor is quite justified in refusing to divulge questions of professional secrecy . . . . The judge might in some cases refuse to commit a medical man for contempt in refusing to reveal confidences. Every case must be governed by particular circumstances, and the ruling of the judge will be the test '. It is submitted that there is nothing in this statement which conflicts with the general principle enunciated in the text. It must be the judge's discretion in each case to say whether in the circumstances he will or will not commit for contempt. If a medical practitioner is informed by a patient that a crime has been committed, it is his duty to communicate with the authorities; see *per* Avory, J., in his charge to the grand jury at Birmingham Assizes (1914), (49 L. Jo. 713). See also *Kitson* v. *Playfair, supra;* and A.B. v. C.D. (1904), 7 F. (Cf. of Sess.) 72. A medical practitioner ought to divulge confidential information if requested to do so by the patient whom it concerns (C. v. C. (1946) 1 All E.R. 562): see title Divorce, Vol. 12."

In essence, according to English law, a medical practitioner is apparently obliged to report to the authorities any information that a crime has been committed even when this knowledge came to him in his professional capacity. (This obligation does not necessarily apply in other countries, e.g. where Roman Dutch law prevails.) Personally I must adhere to the Oath which enjoins me to regard as secret the information gained as a result of a medical consultation. So holy is the trust between doctor and patient that I believe it cannot be broken. On the other hand, if the doctor finds that his patient is insane, a sexual pervert who has criminally assaulted and killed innocent women or is in such a mental state that he is not aware of what he is doing, he should, in my opinion, issue an urgency reception order under the Mental Disorders Act to detain the patient under proper medical care and thus at the same time prevent him from harming others. Finally, the outcome of this conflict between his duty as a citizen and that of a doctor can only be resolved by the practitioner concerned according to his own conscience.

In practice the medical practitioner or specialist is repeatedly asked by an employer for information on the health of his employee. He is anxious to know the real nature of his complaint. He might want this information for a number of reasons. For instance, he may need to replace him and if he knows the severity of the illness he knows whether to make arrangements for a relief. He is often genuine and has the interest of his employee at heart. Nevertheless the doctor must be careful not to disclose anything confidential even if he knows that the employee is making the most of his illness. He must at all costs avoid placing his patient in an embarrassing situation. He should tell the patient that he has been asked for this information and, if he agrees, give him a letter for his employer telling him the nature of the illness and its likely progress.

Under certain circumstances an individual is prepared to reveal his medical history to a particular group. For instance, when he agrees to join a service with a pension scheme such as the government administration, military forces, or a large industrial concern he is obliged to pass a medical test. Once he is accepted the firm will be concerned with his future fitness. If he is absent from work for more than a very short period the reason will be asked and a medical certificate giving the nature of his illness will be expected. If he is absent for longer than a certain period a medical board may be demanded to determine whether he will be fit for future service. Therefore, when accepting employment in such a service the person enters it with the knowledge that this firm or service will wish to know the nature of his previous illnesses. If he refuses to comply he will not be admitted to its ranks. Often the service employs its own doctors who, in its interests, are required to reveal the nature of the employee's disorder. The doctor concerned is not divulging any secret in making available this information to the organisation as the employee has agreed to be examined for this purpose and has completed a form giving details of all his previous illnesses.

Failure to pass on a correct message may cause an error or

mishap. For instance, a wrong or misunderstood telephone communication may result in an incorrect entry on the patient's admission form to the hospital and if the correct diagnosis is not passed on properly a wrong operation may be performed. The recipient of a communication may fail to read the message or forget to pass it on to the right quarters. The doctor is responsible for those he appoints to receive or deliver messages on his behalf and in the case of a medical practitioner his wife is included in this category.[1]

No Pessary to Cause Abortion

Most doctors will agree with me that the question of terminating a pregnancy is a difficult one for the decision depends greatly on the doctor's conscience, which determines his attitude towards this act. And this again is influenced by his religious principles and his medical code. For instance, in the Roman Catholic faith the belief is that no one has the God-given right to directly take a foetal life under any circumstances even though that of the mother may be endangered. Personally, my conscience has been at ease when a pregnancy had to be ended because the life of the mother was threatened or her future health jeopardised by its continuation. I have accepted that if a mother dies as a result of the pregnancy her other children would be denied the care so vital for their upbringing. On the other hand, my conscience does not allow me to agree to prematurely terminating it on social or even vague psychosomatic grounds. For example, poverty, too many children, hardships and anxiety, do not prick my conscience unduly. I am able to refuse such requests. I am more disturbed when an unmarried girl is involved. In this circumstance I find myself wondering what I would do if she were my own daughter. Again I have refused no matter how painful the circumstances were. There follows the even more difficult question of rape. We have heard that in recent Congo riots members of a religious order were raped and so could have become pregnant. Even in this case

[1] *Medical Chronicle* Editorial, November, 1966.

I can see no valid reason for interfering with the natural course of this state although the offence was against the will of the unfortunate women. No insoluble problem was created by such pregnancy. The baby could be expected to be normal at birth and the mother would not necessarily suffer permanent harm. After birth the baby could be cared for very adequately by foster parents. No stigma appears to pertain to the mother in this particular instance since she was completely innocent. The medical point of view appears to be that nobody has the right to directly take the life of a child even if it is in the foetal stage of development, provided it can be shown that the mother's future life is not threatened. The Roman Catholic faith, however, forbids the taking of life directly under any circumstances though in some instances this may happen indirectly. For example, it is permissible to remove a malignant uterus which happens to be gravid at the same time. In such a case the motive is to remove a lethal organ even though its indirect effect is the destruction of the foetus.

I have already stated that the purpose of medicine is to preserve life. Is it unethical to agree to the termination of a pregnancy in the eighth to twelfth week in a mother who has contracted German measles even though her life is in no way endangered? I find this problem hard to resolve. The horror of a blind, deaf or idiotic human being born into this world appals me and I would have the greatest difficulty in condemning a mother to bring forth a child with such an intolerable handicap. It is perhaps asking too much to allow anybody to start his existence without even the potentiality of being able to fend for or defend himself. I have little doubt that even to a Roman Catholic the death of a hydrocephalic monster within hours of birth is a tremendous relief! Yet there are many who would object to killing a foetus in utero with German measles since the chances of a normal baby being born are good. They ask whether there is any difference between this act and euthenasia. I must agree that it is a most difficult matter to decide whether a foetus should be removed because of possible abnormalities.

THE ABORTION ACT 1967

The Abortion Act 1967 [Chapter 87] amends and clarifies the law relating to termination of pregnancy by registered medical practitioners. In effect this Act gives statutory force to certain aspects of the decision in the case of *R. v Bourne* (1939) 1 K.B. 687. In that case it was held that on a prosecution under section 58 of the Offences Against The Person Act 1861, for using an instrument with intent to procure miscarriage, the burden rests on the Crown to prove that the operation was not done in good faith for the purpose only of preserving the life of the mother, and if in the opinion of the jury that burden is not discharged, the accused is entitled to a verdict of acquittal. The learned judge said that the words " preserving the life of the mother " must be construed in a reasonable sense. The law did not require a doctor to wait until the unfortunate woman is in peril of immediate death. Where it is reasonably certain the mother will not be able to deliver the child and survive the doctor is not only entitled, but it is his duty to perform the operation with a view to saving her life. But these words were not limited to the case of saving the mother from death. The judge went on to say (at pp. 693-4) :

" I think those words ought to be construed in a reasonable sense, and, if the doctor is of opinion, on reasonable grounds and with adequate knowledge that the probable consequences of the continuance of pregnancy will be to make the woman a physical or mental wreck, the jury are quite entitled to take the view that the doctor who, under those circumstances and in that honest belief, operates, is operating for the purpose of preserving the life of the mother ".

The legal position is now governed by the provisions of The Abortion Act 1967 and in particular subsections 1 and 2 of section 1 which provide :

" 1. Subject to the provisions of this section, a person shall not be guilty of an offence under the law relating to abortion when a pregnancy is terminated by a registered medical practitioner if two registered medical practitioners are of the opinion, formed in good faith—

(a) that the continuance of the pregnancy would involve risk to the life of the pregnant woman, or of injury to the physical or mental health of the pregnant woman or any existing children of her family, greater than if the pregnancy were terminated; or

(b) that there is a substantial risk that if the child were born it would suffer from such physical or mental abnormalities as to be seriously handicapped.

2. In determining whether the continuance of a pregnancy would involve such risk of injury to health as is mentioned in paragraph (a) of subsection (1) of this section, account may be taken of the pregnant woman's actual or reasonably forseeable environment."

The Act also lays down a certain procedure which is to be followed in carrying out an abortion in reliance on the Act. These aspects include the provision that any treatment for the termination of pregnancy must be carried out in a hospital or in a place approved for that purpose except where such termination " is immediately necessary to save life or to prevent grave permanent injury to the physical or mental health of the pregnant woman." Section 4 provides that a person who has a conscientious objection to participating in this type of treatment is not under any legal compulsion to do so, but this express exception does not relieve him from or affect his common law duty to participate in treatment which is necessary to save life or to prevent " grave permanent injury to the physical or mental health of a pregnant woman ".

It will be observed that section 1(1) permits the termination of pregnancy where, *inter alia,* the continuance of pregnancy involves risk to life or to physical and mental health greater than if the pregnancy were terminated. The use of the word " greater " obviously relates to degree but does not deal with the extent to which such risk must be " greater ". In *Bourne's* case the judge referred to the case where continuance of pregnancy would make her "a physical or mental wreck." This is clearly no longer the test, particularly as the Act refers in relation to where such treatment must be carried out or concerning a conscientious objector, to "grave permanent injury to the physical or mental health of a pregnant woman." The provisions of section 1, therefore, widen the scope within which medical termination of pregnancy is authorised by law. While this would not always be the position, very often her desire or her subjective reasons for the wish to terminate pregnancy could provide the justification for its fulfilment.

It must be emphasised, however, that while the provisions of section 1 have the effect of widening the limits within which abortion is allowed by law, there still exist defined limitations upon the lawful termination of pregnancy. Medical practitioners must give effect to the provisions of the section and in particular to the requirement that the risk to life or injury to physical or mental health must be " greater ". Although it is a matter of degree a doctor must be satisfied that it is " greater " in the sense that in his opinion formed in good faith the termination of pregnancy is justified.

Within recent years it would appear that the public has come to regard a foetus as not an individual with a recognisable personality and therefore its destruction could not carry the same implication for them as has that of the child killed after birth. To me it is murder in both instances. Since environment and social health have long been linked there is now emerging a tendency to cloak social purpose with medical argument.

The highly controversial clause in the 1967 Act is the permitting of an abortion if that birth could adversely affect the physical health of any of the children of that family. To me this would be particularly difficult of proof just as would the impairment of mental health of a mother if pregnant. A doctor ought not be required to make decisions in non-medical grounds, since he is not specially trained to do so. At first sight it might appear to some a relatively simple matter to allow abortion when there is a danger that a gravely defective child will be born. However, in only a very few cases can a doctor diagnose such deformity with any degree of certainty and probably never in the earliest stages of pregnancy. If the intention of the Act of 1967 be to reduce the number of back-street abortions this would be humane in the light of the unfortunate tragedies which have so often followed such practices. This result, however, is by no means certain, nor does it follow that the minority of irresponsible medical practitioners who engaged in such practice before the 1967 Act will cease their activity thereafter since the more affluent may still desire to buy silence.

The Declaration of Helsinki

Following on the Declaration of Geneva the World Medical Congress in 1964 adopted another code of ethics which advises the doctor on his attitude towards human experimentation. It is commonly known as the Declaration of Helsinki. It is to be expected that after laboratory experiments have proved success-ful medical men should be anxious to try out the new remedies on their patients so that the sick may benefit from the scientist's observations. The new code reminds the doctor that his mission is to safeguard the health of his patient. The Declaration of Geneva states, " The health of my patient will be my first consideration." As the legal responsibilities of physicians vary in different countries, the code of Helsinki was adopted as a guide to them. It distinguishes clearly between clinical research in which the object on the patients concerned is therapeutic and clinical research in which its object is purely scientific, that is without therapeutic value to the person undergoing the trial.

The following outline of the code is quoted in full from the British Medical Association *Members Handbook* (1965), p. 56.

1. Basic Principles

1. Clinical research must conform to the moral and scientific principles that justify medical research and should be

based on laboratory and animal experiments or other scientifically established facts.

2. Clinical research should be conducted only by scientifically qualified persons and under the supervision of a qualified medical man.
3. Clinical research cannot legitimately be carried out unless the importance of the objective is in proportion to the inherent risk to the subject.
4. Every clinical research project should be preceded by careful assessment of inherent risks in comparison to foreseeable benefits to the subject or to others.
5. Special caution should be exercised by the doctor in performing clinical research in which the personality of the subject is liable to be altered by drugs or experimental procedure.

2. *Clinical Research combined with Professional Care*

1. In the treatment of the sick person the doctor must be free to use a new therapeutic measure if in his judgment it offers hope of saving life, re-establishing health, or alleviating suffering. If at all possible, consistent with patient psychology, the doctor should obtain the patient's freely given consent after the patient has been given a full explanation. In case of legal incapacity (*Note* : The phrase " legal incapacity " means " incapacity to give consent freely ".) consent should also be procured from the legal guardian; in case of physical incapacity the permission of legal guardian replaces that of the patient.
2. The doctor can combine clinical research with professional care, the objective being the acquisition of new medical knowledge, only to the extent that clinical research is justified by its therapeutic value for the patient.

3. *Non-therapeutic Clinical Research*

1. In the purely scientific application of clinical research carried out on a human being it is the duty of the doctor

to remain the protector of the life and health of that person on whom clinical research is being carried out.

2. The nature, the purpose, and the risk of clinical research must be explained to the subject by the doctor.

3a. Clinical research on a human being cannot be undertaken without his free consent, after he has been fully informed; if he is legally incompetent the consent of the legal guardian should be procured.

3b. The subject of clinical research should be in such a mental, physical and legal state as to be able to exercise fully his power of choice.

3c. Consent should as a rule be obtained in writing. However, the responsibility for clinical research always remains with the research worker; it never falls on the subject, even after consent is obtained.

4a. The investigator must respect the right of each individual to safeguard his personal integrity, especially if the subject is in a dependent relationship to the investigator.

4b. At any time during the course of clinical research the subject or his guardian should be free to withdraw permission for research to be continued. The investigator or the investigating team should discontinue the research if in his or their judgment it may, if continued, be harmful to the individual.

These points are in my opinion extremely important in conducting non-therapeutic clinical research. Pappworth,[1] in his book *Human Guinea Pigs,* makes allegations concerning medical experiments on patients who either have not given their consent or have not understood what the investigation entails including the risks. He also states that drugs have been used which have been absolutely contraindicated. I agree with his opinion that the most basic principle—his principle of equality—is that no experimenter should submit a patient to a

[1] Pappworth, M. H. (1967). *Human Guinea Pigs. Experimentation on Man.* Routledge & Kegan Paul, London.

procedure which he would refuse to have carried out on himself or his family.

In underdeveloped countries, where the masses do not always understand Western medical therapeutic trials, subjects often give their consent believing that the drug tried is of proven value. They are often not told that the drug is given as a pure trial and that there is absolutely no risk although the chances of such are small. The trial, of course, may be reasonable since its value has already been shown by animal experimentation. The utmost care should be taken to ensure that all the subjects are thoroughly aware of what is taking place before they give their consent. I would like to see the introduction of control committees in such countries to supervise the institution of trials on indigenous population by medical scientists. It is important for these trials to take place in such countries as well as in any other part of the world in order to benefit the people in them.

Human Experimentation

While animal experiment involving the loss of life is not contrary to the aims of medicine, any experiment or therapeutic trial on a human being which threatens his life or could harm or impair his health permanently or his well-being should be regarded as opposed to its principles. Trials with drugs are constantly being carried out and surgeons are always devising new operations. As long as the procedure is intended to assist and not to hurt man its practice is justified, provided, of course, the experimenter has good reason to believe that what he has planned is not likely to end in disaster and that the procedure has been explained to the patient or his family and agreement to it obtained. As long as the patient is no worse off for what has been done, the doctor need not have a guilty conscience. When deciding on a procedure which may seem risky, we often have to consider as well the dangers of the disease and whether, if it is left untreated, the patient's end is inevitable. For instance, if a patient has malignant hypertension and after examining him the doctor decides he is not likely to live more than a year

9

or two, it might be permissible to try an operation that seems likely to enhance his chances of recovery. He attempts this hoping to prolong the patient's life and operates with the sincere belief that what he is doing is justified. Should the patient not recover or even deteriorate he need have no bitter regrets. The patient would have died in any event and at least he tried a new procedure which held a reasonable chance of success and which, if it had succeeded, would have given the patient a new lease of life. Thus before undertaking a treatment that may in any way be dangerous he has to think very carefully. For instance, he may be engaged on a particular research project in which he is obliged to try the effect of certain drugs which may have harmful effects. At the same time he has to consider the welfare of the patients entrusted to his care. He has to decide how great a risk is entailed in giving them these drugs and whether it is worth trying them on a series of patients in the hope that at least some of them will be cured. He may wish to use one of the radioactive isotopes which he believes will cure the patients, but at the same time he is faced with the thought that although he may be successful there is a slight danger that some of the patients may develop some serious blood disorder, like leukaemia or aplastic anaemia, perhaps many years later. Despite assurances that the dose is mild and the chances of this happening are remote, his conscience pricks him. He wonders if he would use this treatment on himself or on one of his children. " How do we know that the experts are quite right?" he asks himself. " What if they are wrong or the patient has a predisposition to leukaemia and the treatment may precipitate it?" Yet many such trials are being conducted with these drugs throughout the medical world.

No one can be absolutely sure that a drug is entirely safe even if the chances of anything going wrong are very slight. I have often pondered and been worried about the attitude I should adopt towards the use of radioactive isotopes and even X-rays. Many patients have asked me not to take an X-ray of them as they were afraid that one day they might develop cancer or leukaemia as a result. The doctor has to rely on his own conscience. If he has any doubt he should not use the drug or proceed with any experimental trial until he is satisfied from the evidence available that it is safe. But on the other side, if the patient is so ill that the test or drug under consideration makes his immediate prospects of recovery better he should use it without any qualms about its possible consequences perhaps many years later. He must restore his patient's health at the time by the best means available to him. Thus if an X-ray is needed or a radioisotope indicated he should not hesitate.

Medical research on the living is in fact the pattern of medicine today. It would be wrong to mankind to hinder it or its rightful development. It is necessary as animal experimentation. Both have their place in our fight against disease. Professor L. J. Witts in his review of Dr. Pappworth's book on experiments in man (see *Brit. med. J.* (1967) **1**, 689) points out that an exploitation of experiments on the living has led to real advances in the entire field of medicine. The two best examples perhaps are cardiac surgery and renal haemodialysis. But this resulted in two potentially dangerous situations. The first is the pressure on young clinicians to participate in the studies as part of their training for a later clinical appointment. The second is the growth in the numbers of research workers who hope to devote their lives entirely to clinical investigation. Professor Witts warns that each of these groups may be tempted to perform experiments on the living for the sake of their careers rather than for the good of the patient.

Sir Austin Bradford Hill (1963) in his Marc Daniels Lecture (see *Brit. med. J.* (1967) **1**, 1043) finds it difficult to accept any general code of ethical practice which takes no heed of the varying circumstances of clinical medicine. He argues that there may be special circumstances in which the patient's consent need not or even should not be sought in a controlled trial. He makes the point that there are occasions when it may be impossible for an ill-educated and sick person to fully understand the pros and cons of a new and unknown treatment versus an orthodox and known one. The new treatment would of course be relevant to the patient's disease. The doctor does not always know the pros and cons himself. In such a trial he is wholly or to a very large extent ignorant of the relative values and dangers of one of the treatments. In order to consent to a trial the patient must fully understand what he is being asked to do. But if the selected patient cannot really grasp the entire situation or if his confidence in the judgment of the doctor is upset, then according to Sir Austin, the ethical decision as to whether or not it is correct to include him in the trial lies with the doctor. There are specific and extenuating circumstances for each proposed trial. It is only possible to enumerate broad principles of ethical behaviour but it is doubtful if they can be reduced to precise rules of action which would apply in all cases. I personally would insist that if there is any reasonable risk in any controlled trial the subject must understand to what he is consenting. If he or the family do not agree the new experimental treatment should be withheld.

In 1966 the Royal College of Physicians appointed a committee headed by Sir Max Rosenheim to consider how far supervision of clinical investigation was required. The term included all forms of experiment on man. Broadly speaking there were two kinds of clinical investigation or research. The first has diagnostic or therapeutic relevance to the patient and here there is seldom a serious ethical problem posed and in fact the Committee considered that, at times, the doctor failed in his duty to the patient by not carrying out a relevant experiment. The second kind of investigation, however, presents difficult ethical problems to the individual as its object is to advance knowledge although the patient himself cannot benefit directly. The Committee accepted the Declaration of Helsinki and its recommendations. However, it thought it of special importance that clinical investigation should proceed without unnecessary interference or the imposition of rigid bureaucratic control since this might deter doctors from carrying out investigations which might provide valuable information. The Committee was satisfied that a high ethical standard was maintained in Britain. It recommended that all clinical investigation should be conducted with skill and care and advice sought by even those most experienced. Secondly it suggested that in medical institutions, where clinical investigation is being conducted all projects should be approved by a group of doctors experienced in this field. And in non-medical institutions where clinical experiments are done on man, at least one medically qualified person with experience in clinical investigation should be in the advisory group. The Committee refrained from formulating precise rules for supervision because the way in which this could be achieved varied in different institutions. (See Report of the Committee appointed by the Royal College of Physicians of London. *Brit. med. J.* (1967) **2,** 429.)

The medical profession appreciates the value and justification of animal experimentation. Sir Peter Medawar, F.R.S.,[1] advocated its use for the furtherance of medical knowledge. Realising the opposition to animal experimentation by many of the public and a few of the medical profession as well, he asks medical scientists to reassure people that medical research is being conducted properly, and considers the training of animal technicians does much to lessen criticism against animal experiments. He dismisses ignorant sentimentality and lack of human understanding and defends the use of experimental animals as already its benefits to mankind are very significant. He refers to their great value in assaying drugs and biological substances. The use of animals is essential to help man and if it were stopped widespread harm might result.

[1] Medawar, Sir Peter (1966). *Br. med. J.,* **2,** 1132.

PUBLIC PROTECTION AND THE
MEDICAL COUNCIL

In the middle ages knowledge of medicine was largely confined to the monasteries or religious orders to which the physicians belonged. They carried out a merely superficial examination and were mainly concerned with the diagnosis and prognosis. The apothecary, or rather grocer who knew about herbal remedies, and the barber-surgeon, who knew about baths and certain simple surgical procedures, were deputed to carry out the instructions of the physician. In 1512 in England the slowly developing medical profession was placed under the control of the Church, which also became its licensing body. This control was extended to include midwives and apothecaries as well should they attempt to practise medicine. Anyone found guilty by an ecclesiastical court of any form of bad practice would be inhibited and if necessary excommunicated (R. S. Roberts, personal communication).

During the sixteenth century medical knowledge advanced especially in the fields of anatomy and chemical distillation. With the greater importation of medicine and spices from abroad the apothecary began to play a bigger role in the management of disease. As a result those concerned with this aspect of medicine broke away from the grocers and to protect their interests formed themselves into a medical guild. The same happened to the barber-surgeons and thus arose the United Company of Barber-Surgeons in 1540 and the Society of Apothecaries of London in 1617. The surgeon learned his trade by being apprenticed to a master, hence the word " Mister " used today to designate the surgeon. By this time too the physician was beginning to loosen his contact with the

Church, whose control was not proving to be very effective. He was now a more learned man who took about 14 years to obtain his M.D. degree at Oxford or Cambridge or at one of the foreign universities such as Padua. But the physician still belonged to a privileged class and was rewarded with lands or other advantages. There were, too, all kinds of quacks, herbalists and bone setters. Anyone (including the medical practitioner) could be prosecuted in the King's Court for damages arising out of negligence, but there could be little check on unethical conduct unless deliberate fraud was probable. In order to protect the public from these charlatans and to keep medicine in the hands of properly qualified persons the Royal College of Physicians was founded in 1518 as a body of physicians licensed to practise in London and its immediate neighbourhood. It granted a licenciate (L.R.C.P.) to these men and only admitted the privileged few with a doctorate from one of the universities. It could also expel a member for incontinency. Their object was not really achieved because their fees were so high that poor men turned more and more to the apothecaries, who in 1815 were given the statutory right to examine and licence candidates as general practitioners. In 1745 the surgeons broke away from the barbers and founded, in 1800, the Royal College of Surgeons which granted the M.R.C.S. But as none of these medical corporations undertook the training of doctors medicine hardly advanced under this system.

The real impetus to the development of medicine started in the hospitals like St. Bartholomew's and St. Thomas's which later linked their hospital training with university teaching. Many of the practitioners took the licence of the Society of Apothecaries as well as the M.R.C.S., combining their apprenticeship with walking the wards of the London hospitals.

The greatest stimulus in medical training came from the University of Edinburgh where in the early eighteenth century its hospital began training doctors in modern clinical methods, modelling its teaching on that of the greatest clinical teacher of Europe—Hermann Boerhaave of Leyden (1688-1738). For the first time British doctors were being trained the modern way as general practitioners, for the University of Edinburgh included in its curriculum medicine, surgery and pharmacy, a move that was strongly resisted by Cambridge and Oxford until the middle nineteenth century. Edinburgh's example was followed in London itself a little later by the new University College which had a hospital attached to it.

The Royal College of Physicians in London excluded the new general practitioner. With the Industrial Revolution and the growth of towns these doctors grew in number and influence and began to object to the ancient privileges enjoyed by the old established medical corporations. They also demanded that medical education should be overhauled, that unqualified practitioners should be made illegal and that there should be a proper standard of examination for qualification. The situation was indeed chaotic for about 50 per cent. of doctors had no real education at all. After a struggle lasting 50 years they were able to compel the government to listen to their pleas and as a result the Medical Act of 1858 was passed. This provided a proper standard for medical practice although the medical corporations were left intact. Prior to the Act a number of bodies as well as universities were granting medical qualifications that entitled the holder to practise medicine. There was thus considerable variation in the standards set. But with the new Act and the institution of the General Medical Council with its medical register, the quality of the examinations was raised and the public assured of a good ethical standard of medical practice in Great Britain. Today more and more doctors are seeking a university degree in preference to the diplomas and training of the medical corporations.

It is said that a profession differs from a trade or business in that it is controlled by a self-governing body which ensures that its members follow certain ethical requirements. Medicine has its code of ethics which decrees what a medical man may or may not do and what his relations should be with patients and the public. Personal interests are subordinated to this code of behaviour. There must always be differences of opinion. Some people may wish to see the profession behave in a certain way and others may take an opposite view. Thus there is a give and take and the laws under which a medical council operates were adopted in the first instance after careful consideration by the parliament of each country concerned. They are based on the principles of the Hippocratic Oath and aim at the practice of proper medicine. They stress aspects of this Oath, such as never deliberately harming anyone, using our knowledge and skill for the benefit of the patient, not producing illegal abortions and, above all, never divulging information confided by the patient. Both the Hippocratic Oath and the Geneva Convention emphasise that a doctor must conduct himself in a fitting manner both to the public and the profession which is regarded as a brotherhood of men.

Fundamentally a medical council, in whatever country it is, exists to protect the public against bad or dangerous practice. Therefore to ensure good practice every individual who wishes to serve as a medical practitioner must be accepted on the register of doctors set up by this council. In order to protect the public this body lays down the medical qualifications acceptable to it. Insistence on proper standards of medical education is therefore one of its main functions.

Not only is the medical council concerned with qualifications but it keeps an eye on the members of the profession already admitted and demands that doctors conduct themselves in the correct way whilst practising. For instance practising medicine under the influence of alcohol is viewed very seriously since a practitioner in this state is unlikely to be capable of forming a sound judgment and thus may be deemed negligent. Admittedly we can all recall instances of individuals who are able to practise competently despite consuming large amounts of alcohol. But they are exceptions to the rule. More often when someone is under its influence his judgment is poor and errors result. In order to prove such an offence against a practitioner it must be shown that he has done something wrong during or as a result of his practice. As long as a drunk person is not actually practising medicine in this state the council is not concerned. If a doctor has sexual relations with a woman other than his wife, this is not a matter for the council, provided she is in no way connected with his practice.

Any person who undertakes to give medical advice or treatment expressly or impliedly holds himself out as possessing adequate skill, knowledge and learning for the purpose of carrying out the duties that he undertakes. Such a person, whether he is a registered medical practitioner or not, owes a person who consults him a duty of care. The standard of care and skill to satisfy the duty is that of the ordinary competent medical practitioner. In *R*. v. *Bateman* ((1925) 94 L.J.K.B. 791) Lord Hewart, C. J., said, " If a person holds himself out as possessing special skill and knowledge and he is consulted, as possessing such skill and knowledge, by or on behalf of a patient, he owes a duty to the patient to use due caution in undertaking the treatment. If he accepts the responsibility and undertakes the treatment and the patient submits to his direction and treatment accordingly, he owes a duty to the patient to use diligence, care, knowledge, skill and caution in administering the treatment. No contractual relation is necessary, nor is it necessary that the service be rendered for reward . . . . The law requires a fair and reasonable standard of care and competence . . . . If the patient's death has been caused by the defendant's indolence or carelessness, it will not avail to show that he had sufficient knowledge; nor will it avail to prove that he was diligent in attendance, if the patient has been killed by his gross ignorance or unskilfulness."

Therefore a doctor charged with negligence or sued for damages on the ground of negligence, can clear himself if he shows that he acted in accordance with general and approved practice. He will not be liable in negligence if he acted in accordance with a practice accepted as proper by a responsible body of medical men skilled in that particular art. This means the practice generally approved at the date when he is said to have been negligent and not the practice which gained approval at a later date. Thus an anaesthetist was held not liable when he administered an anaesthetic which had been kept in a manner thought to be safe at the time, which later experience showed to be dangerous. Moreover, a practitioner is not liable for any error or accident; his conduct is judged by the circumstances which prevailed at the time. A mistaken diagnosis is not necessarily a negligent diagnosis. It may be due to a reasonable error of judgment. It is difficult to define with any precision the skill and diligence which a doctor undertakes to furnish in the performance of his obligations to his patients. It is a question of degree and there is a borderland within which it is difficult to say whether a breach of duty has or has not been committed. In the case of *Hatcher v. Black and Ors.* (1954, *The Times,* June 29, 30, July 1, 2), Lord Justice Denning said that no matter what care was used there was always a risk, and it would be wrong and bad law to say that simply because a mishap occurred the doctor was liable. Indeed, it would be disastrous to the community. It would mean that a doctor examining a patient or a surgeon operating at the table, instead of getting on with his work, would be forever looking over his shoulder to see if someone was coming up with a dagger, for an action for negligence against a doctor was like unto a dagger; his professional reputation was as dear to him as his body—perhaps more so. The court must therefore not find him negligent because of one of the risks inherent when an operation actually took place, or because in a matter of opinion he made an error of judgment. He should be found guilty when he had fallen short of the standard of reasonable medical care, when he was deserving of censure (J. P. Eddy on Professional Negligence, pp. 109-10).

In determining the standard of care which a doctor owes his patient, a great many decided cases exist which serve as a guide and as a test. Negligence may consist in failing to obey an urgent summons from a person who has been accepted as a patient, in failing to warn of the dangers of certain treatment and in unskilful or careless treatment of a complaint properly diagnosed. A practitioner is not liable for negligence because of the possible greater skill of another but it is no defence that he did not attain the standards of a careful and competent practitioner. A competent practitioner should know when a case is beyond his skill and thereupon it becomes his duty to call in a more skilful person. Negligence may also consist in failing to make adequate arrangements for a patient, failing to give proper instructions and failing to communicate his findings to others responsible for continuing a patient's treatment.

A practitioner may also be liable in damages if he is negligent in failing to inform a patient of the risks involved in the treatment and if the patient having been so informed would not have consented. But a doctor often has to make quick decisions in circumstances where it is not possible or even advisable to consult his patient. Thus, when a doctor is dealing with a mentally sick man and has a strong belief that his only hope of cure is submission to electro-convulsive therapy, the doctor cannot be criticised if he does not stress the dangers, which he considers to be minimal, which are involved in that treatment (see *Bolam* v. *Friern Hospital Committee* 1957 (2) A.E.R. 118 at p. 124). Generally speaking there is an implied consent by a patient to do what the surgeon without negligence considers necessary or desirable. (See Halsbury's Laws of England 3rd edn. vol. 26 pp. 17-19). It has been held (in *Kenny* v. *Lockwood Clinic Ltd.* 1932 1 D.L.R. 507) that the relationship of a surgeon and patient is one in which trust and confidence must be placed in the surgeon. The duty is cast on the surgeon to deal honestly with the patient as to the necessity, character and importance of the operation and its probable consequences " but such duty does not extend to warning the patient of the dangers incident to, or possible in, any operation, nor the details calculated to frighten or distress the patient " (per HODGINS, J. A.). (See Lord Nathan on Medical Jurisprudence pp. 52-54 and Charlesworth on Negligence 4th edn. paragraphs 1015-18.)

The physician cannot always be in constant attendance upon

his patient, who may have to be left to his own devices; and if the former knows of some specific danger and the possibility of its occurring it may well be part of his duty to his patient to advise him of the proper action in such an emergency. This principle has been adopted in Canada (see *Murrin* v. *James* 1949 D.L.R. 403) and in South Africa (see *Dube* v. *Administrator, Transvaal* 1963 (4) S.A. 260 at p. 269). It accords with the views expressed in many judgments in the United Kingdom. This important aspect is summarised by Lord Nathan in his very useful book on this subject, Medical Jurisprudence, at pp. 46-47, as follows:

" In many cases it is reasonable or even necessary for the medical man to make the patient himself responsible for the performance of some part of the treatment which the medical man has undertaken to give. Where, as often happens, the medical man's course of action depends upon a report by the patient as to his condition or symptoms or as to the progress of the treatment, the medical man has no choice in the matter; he must rely upon the patient for the necessary information by which to determine what action should be taken, and must therefore, in a sense, delegate to the patient part of his own duties. Frequently also it would be quite unreasonable to expect the medical man to be in constant attendance upon the patient or to exercise supervision over every detail of the treatment; he is compelled therefore to delegate to the patient the performance of some part of the treatment or cure. In many cases, for example, he must rely upon the patient to take the medicine or drugs he has prescribed in accordance with his instructions; and sometimes exact compliance with those instructions will be of supreme importance, as where the patient is having insulin treatment for diabetes mellitus.

In all these cases where the medical man justifiably delegates to the patient the performance of some part of the treatment, there is a special duty towards the patient to give clear and unambiguous instructions, to explain to the patient in intelligible terms what is required of him and to give him any warning which may be necessary in the circumstances; and a failure in any of these respects may amount to a breach of duty and expose the medical man to liability for any injury which occurs."

With the phenomenal development of science and its impact on the practice of medicine and with the increase of doctors in a salaried service the intimate or personal links between doctor and patient have tended to grow less. The patient is liable to look upon his medical adviser more as a scientist, one who is an expert and who should know all the latest devices and developments no matter how complicated. Accuracy in scientific data and results are all linked with the modern scientific outlook. Therefore the public are more and more tempted to blame the doctor, nurse or hospital for any unexpected or unfavourable result. The medical practitioner too realises this and always keeps in mind the risks he runs. Very often he is not to blame. It is necessary for him to know what precautions he should take so as not to be caught unawares and to ensure that he is always covered. This is not difficult although he cannot always prevent an attack from an unexpected quarter.

The Doctor Must Not Advertise

Those in practice as well as many of the public appreciate that in Britain a doctor may not advertise his skill in whatever line of medicine he depends for a livelihood. If he is in full-time employment and cannot gain materially from such advertising no harm will come to him. But if it is suspected that he has spoken or let it be known to the outside world, the press, radio or other medium that he has had some special experience in a certain field of medicine, it may well be interpreted that he has used this medium to further his own ends at the expense of his colleagues who also have to earn a living.

Here I would like to quote from the B.M.A. *Handbook,* page 78, on " publicity " as it demonstrates well the attitude of the profession towards this matter.

Publicity

" 4. (i) Anonymity should be observed by the medical profession as a general principle. Departure from this principle is permissible only when the objective of publicity for a doctor or group of doctors is apparent, paramount, and justifiable:

   (a) in the interests of the general public; or

   (b) in the interests of the medical profession; or

   (c) as an essential part of providing authoritative information when necessary for the general public.

In these circumstances anything that could be construed as advertising of the doctor himself should be incidental and reasonably unavoidable for the attainment of the objective.

(ii) Any publicity by or on behalf of or condoned by a doctor which has as its objective the personal advertisement of the doctor is highly undesirable, unethical, and in contravention of paragraph 5 (b) of the Notice of the Disciplinary Committee of the General Medical Council.

(iii) Therefore no active steps should be taken by any registered or provisionally registered medical practitioner to achieve publicity as a doctor except as indicated in paragraph (i) above. A doctor should take all possible steps to avoid or prevent publicity where it can be shown to be unnecessary or to be to his advantage as a doctor.

(iv) Two forms of publicity that are particularly suspect are —frequency of mention of a doctor's name and reference to his being skilled in some particular form of treatment or department of medicine, or in the use of some special apparatus or the performance of some particular operation.

(v) A doctor who attempts to justify unduly frequent publicity on the grounds that it cannot benefit him professionally is doing a disservice in that he makes it more difficult to condemn similar activities on the part of others who do stand to gain thereby.

5. It is conceded that practitioners may properly place their views on medical subjects before the public when they can

[1] British Medical Association (1965). *Members Handbook,* pp. 78 and 79.

do so with authority. In so doing it behoves each one to avoid methods which could be fairly regarded as for the purpose of obtaining patients or otherwise promoting his own professional advantage. It should also be remembered that there are many things innocent in themselves which may, by the manner or frequency of their doing, gravely contravene the principle that medical practitioners should not advertise.

Discussions in the lay press or in broadcasting on controversial points of medical science and treatment should be avoided by practitioners. Such matters are more appropriate to medical journals and for discussion in professional societies."[1]

Men, in my experience, generally resent an individual who boasts about his own skill or ability. Despite the fact that his cult is magical or spiritual, the witchdoctor too does not approve of talking about his prowess as a healer. The witchdoctors I have met do not boast of their skill; they are modest and always maintain that it is for the public to decide on their ability. They believe that only charlatans adopt such an unethical line of approach. I am using this example purely to show how men, uninfluenced by worldly affairs, view this practice which is often referred to rather unfairly as " primitive."

We can understand the reason for the objection to self-advertisement by medical men. If we could be certain that whenever a person boasts of his powers he really possesses this ability no harm would come to the patient. But usually the reverse obtains. Because the doctor finds he is lacking in some aspect of medicine he tries by unfair means to let it be known that he is skilled in the handling of a certain disorder. If this is untrue the unfortunate patient, who places his trust in him, suffers. But not only ignorant and poorly qualified doctors advertise their skill. It is not rare for an able and even more brilliant man to try to gain an unfair advantage over his colleagues. A shrewd yet competent man can be dishonest and when he finds the opportunity of furthering his own ends

[1] British Medical Association (1965). *Members Handbook*, pp. 78 and 79.

seizes the chance to let it be known that he saved a certain person's life when all the other doctors, professors and others had failed. The tragedy of this sort of practice is that although the public may not see through it, members of the medical profession sooner or later learn the source of the information and the doctor concerned loses the respect of his own colleagues. This is perhaps the worst thing that can happen to any doctor.

However there is still much confusion within the ranks of the medical profession as well as the public press as to what constitutes advertising. A doctor may be so afraid of publishing work in the press, lest it be considered advertising, that not infrequently the general public is denied helpful information, since he is too concerned to allow his name or even his discovery to be mentioned. He may be fully entitled to permit his discovery or invention to be quoted but because of his own fears or the jealousy of his colleagues in practice he refuses to allow his contribution to be referred to, even anonymously, lest its source be traced.

As long as the practitioner is not seeking his own personal advantage in order to induce potential patients to seek his services, there is no harm in making available his knowledge to the world. Such concern has been expressed by members of the profession against the use of medical names that the press sometimes avoids mention of medical matters lest it becomes involved in accusations of advertising. If a doctor makes a genuine contribution or is honoured for his services there is no reason for secrecy provided this information is put forward in a purely factual manner. Members of the medical profession should take pleasure in the contributions of their colleagues. A victory for one medical man is a victory for the whole profession. Its status is elevated in the eyes of the outside world.

The General Medical Council of Great Britain

Following on these general remarks about the purpose of a medical council, I think it would be useful to describe in greater detail the functions of the General Medical Council of Great Britain as it affords a good example of what such a body stands for and because it is the one on which many other countries, especially those in the British Commonwealth, have modelled their own.

The General Medical Council is constituted under, and enjoys the powers conferred by, the Medical Act, 1956 (C. 76). It consists of eight members nominated by Her Majesty, twenty-eight appointed members chosen by certain universities and eleven members elected by medical practitioners. The President is elected by the Council from among their number. The Act also provides for the appointment of registrars, secretaries, treasurers and other officers. There are branch councils for England and Wales, for Scotland and for Ireland, to which may be delegated, with certain exceptions, such of the powers and duties vested in the General Council as the Council may see fit.

The General Council's powers and duties include the keeping of a general register and the registrar of each branch council must keep a local register containing qualifications and the addresses and dates of registration of persons registered therein. The Act imposes a duty upon the General Council to secure the standard of proficiency required from candidates at a qualifying examination which is such as " sufficiently to guarantee the possession of the knowledge and skill requisite for the efficient practice of medicine, surgery and midwifery ". For this purpose the General Council is authorised to appoint inspectors to attend all or any of the qualifying examinations held by any of the universities and other bodies specified in the third schedule to the Act. Such inspectors have no right to interfere with the conduct of any examination but it is their duty to report to the General Council " their opinion as to the sufficiency of every examination which they attend and any other matters relating to such examination which the General Council may require them to report." The General Council must forward such a report from an inspector and the observations of the university or body concerning whom the report relates to the Privy Council. The General Council is also entitled to appoint persons to visit medical schools " subject to any directions which the Privy Council may deem it expedient to give and to compliance with any conditions specified in such directions." While such visitors must not interfere with the giving of any instruction, it is their duty to report to the General Council concerning the sufficiency of the instruction given in the places which they visit.

If at any time it appears to the General Council that the course of study or examinations for registrable qualifications are not such as to secure the " requisite knowledge and skill for the efficient practice of their profession " it may make representations to the Privy Council. The Privy Council may in such circumstances order that such insufficient or inadequate course of study or examination shall not be a qualification registrable under the provisions of the Act.

Section 27 of the Medical Act provides that the privileges of registered practitioners include the right to recover fees for services provided by them. There is a presumption at law that a registered medical practitioner renders his services to a patient for reward (see *Corbin* v. *Stewart* (1911) 28 T.L.R. 99). The onus is therefore placed on a patient to prove an agreement that the doctor rendered his services gratuitously.

The question of discipline is dealt with in great detail in the Act. " The Disciplinary Committee " constituted under section 32 of the Act, is entrusted with disciplinary control of medical practitioners.

Once registered, medical practitioners come under the disciplinary jurisdiction granted to the General Council, which, for this purpose, maintains " The Disciplinary Committee " and " The Penal Cases Committee."

Whenever a fully or provisionally registered person is convicted by a court in the United Kingdom or Republic of Ireland of any crime (except minor motoring offences), the Police authorities make a report to the General Council. The Penal

Cases Committee then considers the matter and decides whether it need go for inquiry before the Disciplinary Committee; for in some cases, such as a first conviction for drunkenness it may decide that a letter of warning will suffice. Similarly in the case of any complaint made to the General Council about the conduct of a registered practitioner, the Penal Cases Committee will decide whether an inquiry is necessary.

The Disciplinary Committee then holds the inquiry. This Committee consists of the President and 18 other members of the Council. After due inquiry they may, if they think fit, direct the erasure from the register of the name of the practitioner who has been convicted of crime or who, in the case of one whose conduct was complained of, is judged to have been guilty of infamous conduct in any professional respect. The Committee may also order erasure from the register if it is proved that any entry has been fraudulently or incorrectly made. The Committee also deals with applications for the restoration to the register of the names of practitioners whose names have been erased on the grounds mentioned above. All acts of the Committee must be decided by the votes of a majority of the members present at the meeting. The quorum of the Disciplinary Committee is five. The Committee is responsible for the making of rules as to the times and places of its meetings and the mode of summoning members, and as to the procedure to be followed and the rules of evidence to be observed in the conduct of its proceedings.

For the purpose of advising the Disciplinary Committee on questions of law arising in proceedings before them, provision is made for the appointment of an assessor who must be a barrister, advocate or solicitor of not less than 10 years' standing. The Lord Chancellor may make rules as to the functions of such assessor. The rules of the Committee provide that it may receive any such oral or other evidence as would be receivable in a court of law and generally the nature of evidence which will be admissible before it. The Committee may administer oaths, witnesses may be summoned, it may also deliberate *in camera* with or without the legal assessor, during or after the hearing. Subject to this exception it must hold its proceedings in the presence of the parties and in public, except where on grounds of justice or for any other special reason it appears to the committee that the public should be excluded from any proceedings or part thereof. Any party may appear either in person or be represented by counsel or solicitor or by an officer of an organisation of which he is a member or by any member of his family. Its proceedings may be published in the same manner as those of any quasi-judicial body.

The holding of a due enquiry involves " at least a full and fair consideration of any evidence that the accused desires to offer and, if he tenders them, hearing his witnesses." The Disciplinary Committee must hold an inquiry in accordance with the rules governing its procedure. (See General Medical Council Disciplinary Committee (Procedure) Rules 1958.) But even then there can have been no due inquiry if the rules of natural justice have not been observed. (See *Fox* v. *General Medical Council* 1960 (3) A.E.R. 225 at pp. 227-8.) It has been held in *Bhandari* v. *Advocates Committee* (1956 (3) A.E.R. 742) that in every allegation of professional misconduct involving an element of deceit or moral turpitude, a high standard of proof is called for and a body of professional men sitting in judgment on a colleague would not be content to condemn on a mere balance of probabilities.

An appeal lies against erasure from the register to the Privy Council. Special rules govern the procedure upon such appeals. The sentence of erasure must appear to be wrong and unjustified for the Privy Council to interfere with it. No general test can be laid down for each case must depend entirely on its own particular circumstances. (See *McCoan* v. *General Medical Council* 1964 (3) A.E.R. 143 at p. 147.) The Privy Council also acts on the principle that an appeal must fail unless there was some defect in the conduct of the inquiry, by way of admission or rejection of evidence or otherwise, that might fairly be thought to have been of sufficient significance to the result to invalidate the Disciplinary Committee's decision. (See *Fox* v. *General Medical Council* 1960 (3) A.E.R. at p. 229 and *Sivarajah* v. *General Medical Council* 1964 (1) A.E.R. 504 at p. 507.)

The meaning of the term "infamous conduct in any professional respect" is serious misconduct judged according to the rules written or unwritten governing the profession. (See Scrutton, L. J., in *Rex* v. *General Medical Council* 1930 (1) K.B.D. 562 at p. 569.) In an earlier case (*Allison* v. *General Council of Medical Education and Registration* 1894 (1) Q.B.D. 750), Lopes, L. J., gives the following definition with which Lord Esher, M.R., and Davey, L. J., agree: "If it is shown that a medical man, in the pursuit of his profession, has done something with regard to it which would be reasonably regarded as disgraceful or dishonourable by his professional brethren of good repute and competency," then it is open to the General Medical Council to say that he has been guilty of "infamous conduct in a professional respect." The question is not whether what was done was an infamous thing for anyone else to do but whether it was an infamous thing for a medical practitioner to do. An act which is not done in a professional respect does not come within the definition. (See Halsbury's *Laws of England,* 3rd ed., vol. 26, p. 64 and the *Functions, Procedure and Disciplinary Jurisdiction, General Medical Council, 1967.*) It is obvious that each case will depend on its facts and circumstances and no exhaustive list of modes of conduct or misconduct which will be covered by the provision can be set out or enumerated. With such reservation in mind, the General Medical Council has given examples of types of misconduct which raise disciplinary issues. (See Functions, Procedure and Disciplinary Jurisdiction 1967.) These include, firstly, abuse of a doctor's knowledge or privileges such as by procuring or attempting to procure an abortion or a miscarriage (if done in circumstances which contravene the law) or improperly purveying dangerous drugs. Secondly, abuse of the relationship between doctor and patient, as, for example, committing adultery with a patient or improperly disclosing information obtained in confidence from a patient. Thirdly, disregard of personal responsibilities to patients, such as gross neglect in diagnosis or treatment or assisting unregistered persons to practice medicine. Fourthly, offences indicative of tendencies dangerous to patients as would arise from a conviction based on abuse of alcohol, especially when in charge of motor vehicles, or as a result of a breach of the Dangerous Drug Regulations or some other offence committed by the use of drugs. The fifth category set out in this useful publication relates to offences discreditable to the doctor and his profession and examples given include convictions for false pretences, forgery, fraud, indecent behaviour or assault. Sixthly, issuing untrue or misleading certificates, reports and other documents signed in a professional capacity. The seventh category relates to improper attempts to profit at the expense of professional colleagues by canvassing for patients, advertising or by the depreciation of the professional skill or ability of another doctor. The last example deals with the abuse of financial opportunities afforded by medical practice. Examples of this include improperly obtaining money from patients or from authorities under the National Health Service, fee-splitting or improperly prescribing drugs or appliances in which a doctor has a financial interest.

The examples given of what could constitute infamous conduct, while not exhaustive, do serve as a useful guide to practitioners in their conduct and behaviour in a professional capacity and are based, as the publication of the General Medical Council says, on its experience over the last 100 years. It may be pointed out that complaints that practitioners have been guilty of infamous conduct, or allegations that entries have been fraudulently or incorrectly made, can be referred to the Penal Cases Committee for investigation. This committee or the findings of this committee will determine whether complaints or allegations should be referred to the Disciplinary Committee for inquiry. (See Halsbury's *Laws of England* (*supra*) pp. 56, 65 and 70.)

In addition to the control of discipline, by the erasure from or restoration of names to the register and the other duties of the General Medical Council to which reference has been made, there are other duties imposed on the Council by the Act. These include medical education, the appointment of examiners to assist at the examinations held for the purpose of granting primary or additional qualifications, the right to sanction combined examinations to be conducted by any two or more universities and other bodies, and registration of Commonwealth and foreign practitioners. The General Council must also cause to be published under their direction new editions of the British Pharmacopoeia, containing such descriptions of and standards for and such notes and other matter relating to medicines, preparations, materials and articles used in the practice of medicine, surgery or midwifery, as the Council may direct. It is important to note that the Council is not a trade union and it does not exist for the purpose of protecting medical practitioners. The nature of the duty imposed on the Council is to protect the public by ensuring that doctors are properly qualified, that they perform their services to patients with skill and diligence and observe high moral and ethical standards. In so doing, medical practitioners derive a clear advantage by being properly trained and being members of a profession which serves the public efficiently, skilfully, honestly and honourably. In the discharge and in the fulfilment of its own responsibilities the General Council is subject to powers conferred on the Privy Council. So that, if it appears to the Privy Council that the General Council ought to appoint assistant examiners as provided by the Act, or have failed to secure the maintenance of a sufficient standard of proficiency at examinations or ought to exercise any power or duty or to do any act which the Council is obliged to do, the Privy Council may notify their opinions to the General Council. If the

General Council fails to comply with any directions of the Privy Council in these circumstances, then the latter may themselves give effect thereto and for that purpose may exercise any power or do any act or thing which the General Council is authorised to do.

10

ETHICAL STANDARDS

The Ethical Standards Laid Down by the British Medical Association

BESIDES THE more legal description of medical ethics by the General Medical Council, the British Medical Association, which since its foundation in 1832 has made available its rich experience in problems of medical ethics, has a standing committee which confines itself to medical ethics and has created its own " ethical machinery " to resolve disputes between its members. Its attitude towards several of the more important ethical matters is worth discussing.

Professional Confidence

The British Medical Association regards professional confidence as the non-disclosure of information gained by the doctor in the course of his relationship with the patient, such information to be divulged only with the latter's consent, preferably in writing. In 1959 this principle was expressed as follows (see B.M.A. *Members Handbook* (1965) p. 60):—

" It is a practitioner's obligation to observe strictly the rule of professional secrecy by refraining from disclosing voluntarily without the consent of the patient (save with statutory sanction) to any third party information which he has learnt in his professional relationship with the patient.

" The complications of modern life sometimes create difficulties for the doctor in the application of this principle, and on certain occasions it may be necessary to acquiesce in some modification. Always, however, the overriding consideration must be the adoption of a line of conduct that will benefit the patient, or protect his interests."

The State cannot demand information about his patient from a practitioner except through some statutory requirement, such as notification of an infectious disease. He can also be requested by the presiding judge, when under oath in a court of law, to divulge confidential information regarding e.g. criminal acts or venereal diseases but may prefer to serve a term of imprisonment rather than break his ethical code.

The Doctor's Practice

On the important subject of setting up in general practice the British Medical Association is concerned mainly with the doctor who, in the capacity of *locum tenens,* assistant or partner enters into an arrangement with a practitioner already in practice. Usually the principal draws up an agreement with the junior whereby the latter is prevented from practising on his own within a defined area for an agreed period. Once this restrictive document is signed there can be no argument in favour of the *locum tenens,* assistant or partner if he wishes to set up practice in competition with the other doctor at the close of his contract with him. Even if there is no legal agreement between the two parties, the British Medical Association maintains that there is an ethical obligation on the part of a doctor not to affect or reduce the practice of a colleague with whom he was recently engaged in a professional association, unless the written consent of the principal, partner or partners has been obtained. A doctor who has acted as an assistant or a locum tenens for that principal or as a member of a partnership should not set up in the principal's or partner's area of practice, nor should one who has unsuccessfully negotiated for a partnership with him nor indeed one who has made enquiries with regard to such a partnership. To do so would be looked upon as an unethical procedure.

I might enlarge upon this theme by quoting the words of this Representative Body as written in 1925:—(see B.M.A. *Members Handbook* (1965) p. 61). "As a locum tenens is introduced in confidence to the practice of which he/she takes charge, it must be presumed on principles of common equity that he cannot without dishonour commence practice in the neighbourhood where he has acted unless with a written consent obtained either from the practitioner whose substitute he has been, or from the legal representatives of this practitioner. There may, however, be circumstances, for example, the lapse of time, which would make the strict application of this rule an unreasonable interference with the freedom of a practitioner who had acted as a locum tenens. If any such plea for the relaxation of the rule in any individual case can be advanced, the facts should be stated to the Central Ethical Committee and the judgment of the Central Ethical Committee of the point should be accepted as final.'

Personally I am not convinced that it is always unethical for a locum tenens (with no restrictive agreement) to set up in competitive practice at the conclusion of the appointment he has just held in a certain area. It may not be wise as he is liable to upset the doctor who had encouraged him. Relations are bound to be strained and the practitioner is likely to take legal proceedings or other measures to prevent his erstwhile locum from practising in his area. But there may be exceptional circumstances, for a locum tenens may have been tempted into practice with a specific promise of or a view to partnership. In fact the principal has no intention of selling a share. All he wants is some help with his practice and as soon as the junior has completed his period of assistanceship he finds that either the price for the partnership is prohibitive or simply that a partner is not wanted and the principal engages another doctor to work for him with the same bait. It is to his advantage to find a keen willing young medico to whom he can pay a comparatively low salary. His purpose is clear. Under such circumstances, when the junior doctor realises what has happened he becomes defiant and elects to set up in opposition. Just as a locum tenens may be dishonourable at times so it must be admitted that every now and then a principal with unethical aims succeeds in finding an innocent and unsuspecting assistant.

Again much depends on the growth and development of the area in which the locum tenens served. Let us imagine he worked (with no restrictive covenant) in a town or city which is growing so rapidly that he is unlikely to take away any of his principal's practice—indeed there is so much of it that the principal cannot even hope to take on more patients. In such instances we cannot agree that the locum tenens is acting unethically provided he starts in an entirely new area or suburb and far removed from his former employer. He may be rendering a good service to the community by bringing his medical skill to an under-doctored area. On the other hand, if the place in which he served shows no signs of growth and is unlikely to develop further it would be wrong for him to settle there as he would raise such opposition that peaceful relations with his colleague would be impossible and he would find it difficult to practise good medicine.

Every junior, before agreeing to offer his services to any practice in a temporary capacity, must weigh the pros and cons very carefully. He must realise that if he should decide later to settle in this part ill-feeling must result unless he can come to an amicable settlement with the principal of the practice. He must not be tempted by vague offers of shares in the practice. This is such a vital matter in his career that it would be a wise precaution for him to discuss it first with an experienced and trusted person. When a doctor enters another's practice he cannot know how the " partnership " will work. So much depends on the compatibility of temperament and the personal regard between the two parties, and this can only be known after they have worked together for some time.

Notices

The British Medical Association discusses the procedure to be adopted by a practitioner who wishes to make a formal announcement about his practice to his patients or colleagues. A change of address or consulting hours should be announced in a circular letter or by telephone to the patients on his books or by a suitable notice in his waiting room. The lay press must not be used for such an announcement.

A consultant starting a practice in a new place must avoid making any public pronouncement of this fact. He may, of course, let medical practitioners know either through personal contact or by a suitable notice in the medical press. When a doctor intends setting up in general practice in a town or certain area he may wish to advise his colleagues of this fact. This is wise. If he so desires be may call upon the practitioners already established there or send a personal introduction to those doctors likely to be interested. A doctor can seldom practise entirely on his own. Inevitably occasions arise when he has to call suddenly upon another doctor for help, as for instance in the event of illness or the need to leave his practice unexpectedly for a few days. In the interests of both his patients and himself every doctor must establish good relations with his colleagues. This may not be easy because of differences in personality and background but it is usually possible to find one or more colleagues who can be called upon when required or *vice versa* will be grateful for such help from the new doctor. In my view, it is not essential for the newcomer to call on every doctor in the district unless he wishes to do so. In some towns or cities this is virtually impossible because of the large number of practitioners there. Perhaps it is better slowly to develop good and friendly relations with colleagues instead of rushing into hasty arrangements with anyone. By proceeding more gradually and by trial and error a doctor comes to know to whom he may entrust his confidence and his practice. Man being as he is, it is virtually impossible to work in perfect harmony with every colleague and impossible to expect this ideal of every doctor.

Door Plates

So as to avoid any hint of advertising unfairly, ostentatious door plates to the doctor's rooms or surgery should be avoided. The door plate should merely mention his name, qualifications and surgery hours. There is no objection to including higher qualifications on the plate. The same form of entry is permitted in the telephone directory. A local directory may include the doctor's name provided there is a list of other practitioners in the area.

The Doctor and His Colleagues

Sooner or later, and more likely sooner, every practitioner needs to call in a consultant for his patients. The request may come from the patient or his family or the doctor himself may wish to do this. The whole subject of consultation is a most difficult and emotional one. The request may be unnecessary or indeed even unwise in the patient's interest and it is impossible to dictate to a practitioner what he should do in such an event. He may be justified in refusing to call in a consultant. Usually, however, in the patient's interests he agrees to ask for another opinion.

The practitioner has every right to ask whatever colleague he wishes to see the patient and usually has his way. But the patient not uncommonly suggests someone of whom the practitioner disapproves and may even decline to call on unreasonable grounds. He may have a personal reason for not wanting a particular consultant and will not agree to his being admitted to the patient. Experience has taught me that this is usually unwise. It is far better to acquiesce than to refuse merely on personal grounds. By refusing what may be a reasonable request the practitioner lays himself open to criticism, particularly if the patient takes a turn for the worse, and not uncommonly his attitude is resented by the patient who seeks another practitioner.

It is always better for the practitioner to contact the consultant personally about the case and tell him the reason for the consultation. Unfortunately this is not always done. The practitioner may agree, often unwillingly, to the consultation but tells the patient to contact the consultant himself. This is not satisfactory. Clearly the consultant is placed in an awkward position when he has only the word of the patient that the doctor has consented to a consultation. Is he to refuse to see the patient? For a long time I have thought about what action he should take. He might phone the practitioner to confirm what the patient has said. This is probably the best procedure. On the other hand, the practitioner may be difficult to contact. He may be away for a day or two or he may on previous occasions have indicated his resentment when a patient has mentioned that particular consultant's name. He may have repeatedly refused to contact him. If such circumstances are known to the consultant, I can see no reason for him to refuse to see the patient, but, after the consultation, he must write to the practitioner or contact him on the telephone to give his findings and advice. He may receive an unfriendly response, but no matter. At times the consultant may find that the practitioner has refused to attend to the patient any longer. In such a situation he must at once see the patient and the practitioner and try to restore their good relations. If he is unable to mend the breach he must see that the patient is under the care of another practitioner of the patient's own choice.

Much is said about how to conduct a consultation, even who should walk into the room first and who should leave the patient first. There is no doubt that when circumstances permit an ideal consultation is a stimulating experience, but more often that remains a wish. Not uncommonly the consultant finds the diagnosis incorrect or the treatment wrong. He is thus in an embarrassing situation. By imparting this information he may ruin the patient's trust in his practitioner; by not telling him he is denying him the truth and after all it is the patient whose welfare matters. The consultation often takes place in the patient's bedroom and with one or more of his relatives standing by waiting anxiously. Medical etiquette demands that the two doctors leave the patient and the consultant gives his views to the practitioner privately in another room. Then the practitioner either alone or in the presence of the consultant should see the patient and tell him what the latter has found. If he is not convinced about the latter's advice he is free to tell the patient. He may have made a wrong diagnosis or given poor advice. But again this procedure is not always possible. I have found it best, when the practitioner is correct and I agree with all he has done, to express my approval and confidence in his treatment to the patient then and there. This method is most successful. The truth has been told, and the practitioner is pleased that he has managed the case so well. On the other hand, if I find that something has been overlooked or I am not sure of some point I avoid discussing it in front of the patient but ask for a private interview with the practitioner in a quiet part of the house. Here I put my point of view. This procedure works well and the practitioner appreciates the handling of the situation. We agree about what is to be said to the patient if a new line of treatment is to be introduced or another opinion, surgical or otherwise, to be sought. In this way the patient's interests remain paramount.

The medical practitioner should always be able to anticipate the need for a consultation. It is his duty to remember that other opinions should be sought when the patient is not progressing as he should if the diagnosis is in doubt. I often see a good practitioner falter in this part of his work. He feels that if he asks for a second opinion his patient may think less of him. But in the long run it always pays and a doctor who understands human nature will know the right time to call in a colleague.

In certain parts of the world we still see a number of doctors in a partnership in which the division between specialist and general practitioner is not as clear as in a modern city, where the two functions are completely separated, the practitioners referring their patients to consultants with whom they have no special association. The partners work as a group which has

11

its advantages. When one partner is away, busy or on leave one of the others can step into the breach, answer a call or take care of his patients until his return. As a further extension of this association, it often happens that one of the partners, who is particularly interested in midwifery, for example, tends to confine himself to this branch, whilst the others concentrate on the other aspects of practice. And as a further extension of the idea, one or more of the partners move into the surgical or orthopaedic fields and before long a combine of doctors is created, offering a very wide, comprehensive and often competent service to their patients. Doctors not in the combine often look askance at this type of practice, since they feel its members tend to refer all their surgical cases to their own partners and, it is argued, this is dangerous as it might encourage them to look for surgical material to increase the total income of the firm. It is an inherent tendency to restrict the freedom of choice of doctor and patient. Further, a large combine is liable to have too powerful a say in the medical affairs of the town and thus to exert undue influence on its medical policy. This is resented by the doctors who practise singly or in small parnterships. On the whole large " combines" of doctors in private practice are not popular within the ranks of the profession, although their patients may be well content with the services they provide.

Here it is well to quote in full the advice of the Central Ethical Committee of the British Medical Association as formulated in 1950, although some of the points differ a little from what I find satisfactory as a result of my own experience (B.M.A. *Members Handbook* (1965), p. 65) :

" 1. A practitioner consulted is a practitioner who, with the acquiescence of the practitioner already in attendance, examines a patient under this practitioner's care and, either at a meeting of the two practitioners or by correspondence, co-operates in the formulation of diagnosis, prognosis, and treatment of the case. The term ' consultation ' means such a co-operation between practitioners. In domiciliary consultations it is desirable that both practitioners should meet and in other circumstances similar arrangements should obtain wherever practicable.

" 2. It is the duty of an attending practitioner to propose a consultation where indicated, or to acquiesce in any *reasonable* request for consultation, expressed by the patient or his representatives.

" 3. The attending practitioner should nominate the practitioner to be consulted, and should advise accordingly, but he should not unreasonably refuse to meet a registered medical practitioner selected by the patient or by the patient's representatives, although he is entitled, if such is his opinion, to urge that the practitioner selected has not the qualifications or the experience demanded by the particular requirements of the case.

" 4. The arrangements for consultation should be made or initiated by the attending practitioner. The attending practitioner should ascertain in advance the amount of the fee, if any, to be paid to the practitioner consulted, and should inform the patient or his representatives that this should be paid at the time of the consultation.

" 5. In cases where the consultant and the attending practitioner meet and personally examine the patient together, the following procedure is generally adopted and should be observed, unless in any particular instance there is substantial reason for departing from it:

(a) All parties meeting in consultation should be punctual, and if the attending practitioner fails to keep the appointment, the practitioner consulted, after a reasonable time, may examine the patient, and should communicate his conclusions to the attending practitioner in writing and in a sealed envelope.

(b) If the consultation takes place at the patient's residence, the attending practitioner should, on entering the room of the patient, precede the practitioner consulted, and after the examination the attending practitioner should be the last to leave the room.

(c) The diagnosis, prognosis, and treatment should be discussed by the practitioner consulted and the attending practitioner in private.

(d) The opinion on the case and the treatment as agreed should be communicated to the patient or the patient's representatives where practicable by the practitioner consulted in the presence of the attending practitioner.

(e) It is the duty of the attending practitioner loyally to carry out the measures agreed at, or after, the consultation. He should refrain from making any radical alteration in these measures except upon urgent grounds or after adequate trial.

" 6. If for any reason the practitioner consulted and the attending practitioner cannot examine the patient together, the attending practitioner should send to the practitioner consulted a brief history of the case. After examining the patient, the practitioner consulted should forward his opinion, together with any advice as to treatment, in a sealed envelope addressed to the attending practitioner. He should exercise great discretion as to the information he gives to the patient or to the patient's representatives and, in particular, he should not disclose to the patient any details of any medicaments which he has advised.

" In cases where the attending practitioner accepts the opinion and advice of the practitioner consulted he should carry out the measures which have been agreed between them; where, however, the attending practitioner finds he is in disagreement with the opinion and advice of the practitioner consulted he should by suitable means communicate his disagreement to the practitioner consulted.

" 7. Should the practitioner consulted and the attending practitioner hold divergent views, either on the diagnosis or on the treatment of the case, and should the attending practitioner be unwilling to pursue the course of action advised by the practitioner consulted, this difference of opinion should be communicated to the patient or his representatives by the practitioner consulted and the attending practitioner jointly, and the patient or his representatives should then be advised either to choose one or other of the suggested alternatives or to obtain further professional advice.

Note. In the following circumstances it is especially desirable that the attending practitioner should endeavour to secure consultation with a colleague:—

(a) When the propriety has to be considered of performing an operation or of adopting some course of treatment which may involve considerable risk to the life of the patient or may permanently prejudice his activities or capacities, and particularly when the condition which it is sought to relieve by this treatment is not itself dangerous to life;

(b) When any procedure likely to result in death of a foetus or of an unborn child is contemplated, especially if labour has not commenced;

(4) When continued administration of any drug of addiction is deemed desirable for the relief of symptoms of addiction;

(d) When there is reason to suspect that the patient (i) has been subjected to an illegal operation, or (ii) is the victim of criminal poisoning or criminal assault.

" 8. Arrangements for any future consultation or additional investigation should be effected only with the foreknowledge and co-operation of the attending practitioner.

" 9. The practitioner consulted should not attempt to secure for himself the care of a patient seen in consultation. It is his duty to avoid any word or action which might disturb the confidence of the patient in the attending practitioner. The practitioner consulted should not communicate with the patient or the patient's representative subsequent to the consultation except with the consent of the attending practitioner.

" 10. The attending practitioner should carefully avoid any remark disparaging the skill or judgment of the practitioner consulted.

" 11. Except by mutual consent the practitioner consulted shall not supersede the attending practitioner during the illness with which the consultation was concerned.

Acceptance of Patients

A very real problem to every practitioner is the patient who wishes to change to him after already being examined by another doctor. No practitioner should accept anyone whom he understands or knows to be under the care of another doctor. He must communicate with that practitioner immediately, pointing out that he has no wish to take the patient without his consent. The Representative Body of the British Medical Association in 1957 and 1963 enumerated the occasions under which a practitioner ought not to accept a colleague's patient without his consent (B.M.A. *Members Handbook* (1965), p. 67) :

" 1. Any patient or member of a patient's household whom he has previously attended either as a consulting practitioner or as a deputy for a colleague.

" 2. Any patient or member of the patient's household whom he has attended within the previous two years in the capacity of assistant or locum tenens.

" 3. Any patient who at the time of the application is under active treatment by a colleague, unless he is personally satisfied that the colleague concerned has been notified by the patient or his representatives that his services are no longer required.

" 4. Any patient who so applies because his regular medical attendant is temporarily unavailable. In such case he should render whatever treatment for the time being may be required, and should subsequently notify the patient's regular attendant of the steps he has taken.

" Notwithstanding paragraph (3) above, when a practitioner in whatever form of practice is asked for advice or treatment by a patient and has reason to believe that the patient is already under medical care and that the request is made without the knowledge of the attending practitioner, it is the duty of the practitioner so approached to urge the patient to permit him to communicate with the attending practitioner. Should the patient refuse this proposal and *if the circumstances are exceptional* the practitioner is at liberty to examine the patient and to tell the patient his finding and conclusions, but, save for any emergency which exists, he shall not accept the patient for treatment.

"A practitioner, in whatever form of practice, should take positive steps to satisfy himself that a patient who applies for treatment or advice is not already under the active care of another practitioner, before he accepts him."

In general it is unwise to be dogmatic. I would suggest that if a patient under treatment by another doctor insists that he no longer wishes to return to his practitioner, the doctor should first see or telephone this colleague to learn his point of view. Tense as is the situation he will generally agree to his taking over the case. On the other hand, if a patient is no longer undergoing a course of treatment and the doctor is satisfied that he is at liberty to go elsewhere he is free to accept him. Again, if at any time a doctor becomes aware that a patient is dissatisfied with his services and he doubts whether he can retain him, it is wise to indicate that he has no objection to his seeking care elsewhere. He thus keeps the goodwill of the patient who not uncommonly returns to him some time later. The clinician must keep the peace and avoid a state of tension between himself and the patient. It is in this way that the understanding doctor comes to the fore.

Dichotomy

The secret division of fees by two doctors on a basis of commission is highly improper, even though some doctors practise it without apparently seeing anything dishonest about it. Dichotomy takes place mostly between the surgeon and the general practitioner, probably because surgical fees are so much greater than those of the physician and the surgeon can afford to give some of his earnings to the doctor who introduced the case. A danger with dichotomy is that the general practitioner is tempted to encourage his patients to undergo an operation when there is little indication for it.

Another method of dichotomy between a surgeon and a general practitioner, although not acknowledged as such, is for the former to pay the latter an assistant's fee for helping him at the operation although his assistance is not necessary, unless the patient specifically requests his general practitioner to be present at his operation even though the practitioner knows that his presence is not technically necessary. Some practitioners do not even attend the operation despite receiving the cheque. The practitioner may square his conscience by convincing himself that the fee he receives is not dichotomy but one earned in return for a service. Thus it is difficult to prove the existence of this practice. But once it starts in a town it becomes difficult to eradicate or even control. It tends to spread since other surgeons feel obliged to play the same " game " in order not to lose their practice.

Attendance on Colleagues

It is the custom for doctors in Great Britain and her former colonies not to charge for attention to another medical man or his dependents. This is because of a feeling of unity amongst all members of the profession, an understanding or link between them that is difficult to define. The World Medical Association speaks of a single brotherhood or bond of fellowship that exists amongst all members of the profession no matter where they qualify. Thus it would seem correct or certainly a fine gesture for a medical man not to charge doctors or anyone depending on them. The British Medical Association advises its members to make every effort to retain the traditional practice, whereby attendance by one doctor on another or his dependents is undertaken without a direct charge. It is worth noting that this assistance is restricted to those who depend on the doctor for their support and is therefore not applicable to his parents if they support themselves. This practice is often extended to members of the clergy and their families and to missionaries. This is a personal decision, but as healing in many minds has a religious flavour, this consideration receives the approbation of most doctors.

On the other hand there are those who do not agree that a doctor and his dependents should not be charged for services rendered. Their argument is that each one has to earn his own livelihood and it is thus better not to be beholden to anyone for services rendered to them. Others again would not charge a doctor on the same register as themselves practising in the same country, but consider it permissible to make a fee for those from a foreign territory. Again there is a substantial number of doctors whose services are much sought after by medical men and their families and thus a considerable amount of their time must be spent on this type of work which is being done gratis. However it is more than likely that they are given a token of appreciation for what they do.

Some doctors would prefer to pay their colleagues and meet all expenses incurred for treatment rather than feel obligated to them. They would rather be independent. However the general feeling favours the offering of whatever medical assistance one can to a colleague in distress.

The waiving of fees to medical colleagues generally applies to nurses in actual practice as well. It is the rule rather than the exception not to charge a nurse, especially one who works in a local hospital or clinic or even in a service far removed from the town in which the doctor practises. Doctors accept this attitude because nurses also tend the sick and are thus in a similar position to themselves.

INDEX

Printed by The Central Press (Aberdeen) Ltd.